Study Guide to Accompany

THIRD EDITION

Clinical Nursing Skills

Nursing Process Model
Basic to Advanced Skills

Sandra F. Smith, RN, MS
President, National Nursing Review
Los Altos, California

Donna J. Duell, RN, MS
Director of Nursing
Cabrillo College
Aptos, California

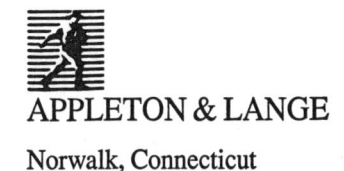

APPLETON & LANGE
Norwalk, Connecticut

0-8385-1365-4

Notice: The authors and the publisher of this volume have taken care that the
information and recommendations contained herein are accurate and compatible
with the standards generally accepted at the time of publication. Nevertheless,
it is difficult to ensure that all the information given is entirely accurate
for all circumstances. The publisher disclaims any liability, loss, or damage
incurred as a consequence, directly or indirectly, of the use and application
of any of the contents of this volume.

Copyright © 1992 by Appleton & Lange
Simon & Schuster Business and Professional Group

All rights reserved. This book, or any parts thereof, may not be used
or reproduced in any manner without written permission. For information,
address Appleton & Lange, 25 Van Zant Street, East Norwalk, Connecticut, 06855.

92 93 94 95 96 / 10 9 8 7 6 5 4 3 2 1

Prentice-Hall International (UK) Limited, *London*
Prentice-Hall of Australia Pty. Limited, *Sydney*
Prentice-Hall Canada Inc., *Toronto*
Prentice-Hall Hispanoamericana, S.A., *Mexico*
Prentice-Hall of India Private Limited, *New Delhi*
Prentice-Hall of Japan, Inc., *Tokyo*
Simon & Schuster Asia Pte. Ltd., *Singapore*
Editora Prentice-Hall do Brasil, Ltda., *Rio de Janeiro*
Prentice Hall, *Englewood Cliffs, New Jersey*

Editor in Chief: Barbara Ellen Norwitz
Production Editor: Elizabeth Ryan

PRINTED IN THE UNITED STATES OF AMERICA

Contents

Introduction v

SECTION I. REVIEW QUESTIONS 1

Chapter One. Professional Nursing 3
Chapter Two. Nursing Process 5
Chapter Three. Patient Care Management 7
Chapter Four. Documentation 9
Chapter Five. Communication and Relationship Skills 11
Chapter Six. Safe Patient Environment 13
Chapter Seven. Bathing and Bedmaking ...15
Chapter Eight. Personal Hygiene 17
Chapter Nine. Vital Signs 19
Chapter Ten. Body Mechanics and Positioning 23
Chapter Eleven. Exercise and Ambulation 25
Chapter Twelve. Admission and Discharge 29
Chapter Thirteen. Basic Physical Assessment 31
Chapter Fourteen. Infection Control and AIDS Care 35
Chapter Fifteen. Medication Administration 37
Chapter Sixteen. Pain Management 41
Chapter Seventeen. Nutritional Management 43
Chapter Eighteen. Specimen Collection 47
Chapter Nineteen. Diagnostic Tests 49
Chapter Twenty. Urine Elimination 53
Chapter Twenty-one. Bowel Elimination 57

Chapter Twenty-two. Heat and Cold Therapy 61
Chapter Twenty-three. Wound Care 65
Chapter Twenty-four. Respiratory Care 67
Chapter Twenty-five. Circulatory Maintenance 71
Chapter Twenty-six. Intravenous Therapy 75
Chapter Twenty-seven. Orthopedic Measures 79
Chapter Twenty-eight. Operative Care 83
Chapter Twenty-nine. Patient Education and Discharge Planning 87
Chapter Thirty. Crisis and the Dying Patient 89
Chapter Thirty-one. Advanced Skills in Nursing Practice 91
Chapter Thirty-two. Home Care 93

SECTION II. STUDY EXERCISES 95

Chapter One. Professional Nursing 97
Chapter Two. Nursing Process 99
Chapter Three. Patient Care Management ..101
Chapter Four. Documentation 103
Chapter Five. Communication and Relationship Skills 105
Chapter Six. Safe Patient Environment 107
Chapter Seven. Bathing and Bedmaking ...109
Chapter Eight. Personal Hygiene 111
Chapter Nine. Vital Signs 113
Chapter Ten. Body Mechanics and Positioning 115

Chapter Eleven. Exercise and
  Ambulation 117
Chapter Twelve. Admission and
  Discharge 119
Chapter Thirteen. Basic Physical
  Assessment 121
Chapter Fourteen. Infection Control
  and AIDS Care 123
Chapter Fifteen. Medication
  Administration 125
Chapter Sixteen. Pain Management 127
Chapter Seventeen. Nutritional
  Management 129
Chapter Eighteen. Specimen Collection 131
Chapter Nineteen. Diagnostic Tests 133
Chapter Twenty. Urine Elimination 135
Chapter Twenty-one. Bowel Elimination ... 137

Chapter Twenty-two. Heat and Cold
  Therapy 139
Chapter Twenty-three. Wound Care 141
Chapter Twenty-four. Respiratory Care 143
Chapter Twenty-five. Circulatory
  Maintenance 145
Chapter Twenty-six. Intravenous
  Therapy 147
Chapter Twenty-seven. Orthopedic
  Measures 149
Chapter Twenty-eight. Operative Care 151
Chapter Twenty-nine. Patient Education
  and Discharge Planning 153
Chapter Thirty. Crisis and the Dying
  Patient 155
Chapter Thirty-one. Advanced Skills in
  Nursing Practice 157
Chapter Thirty-two. Home Care 159

Introduction

This *Study Guide* is designed to be used with the text *Clinical Nursing Skills*, 3rd edition. The desired outcome of the learning process is mastery over a body of knowledge. The wide range of skills and complexity of information contained in the text book, *Clinical Nursing Skills*, necessitate a variety of teaching methods to enhance the learning process. The purpose of this Study Guide is to enable the student to review critical content, identify sections of material that may need further review, and prepare for unit tests, midterms, and final examinations.

The *Study Guide* is divided into chapters and follows the same format as the text. It is divided into two sections. Section I contains Review Questions—questions that focus the student on critical skill content. Written in multiple-choice, true-false, or matching format, these questions are followed by answers with rationale for the correct response to enhance learning. Section II, Study Exercises, provides a guideline for mastering content. The questions in this section are short answer, fill-in, and completion of learning activities. This type of question requires the student to recall, apply, and integrate knowledge. These questions are referenced back to the text for easy access in reviewing the content.

Learning and preparing for tests take place in many ways. Some students are more comfortable taking notes as they read the chapter. Other students highlight key words or phrases and review those areas as their study schema. Whichever study method the student chooses, the *Study Guide* can provide direction for that type of study. In addition, whether the student chooses to study individually or in group sessions, the *Study Guide* can facilitate learning.

The most appropriate use of this *Study Guide* is to follow these guidelines.

- Read the chapter objectives for the assigned chapter(s) in the textbook.

- Read and study the chapter(s) content.

- Verbally or in writing answer the learning objectives.

- Answer the review questions and study exercises in the *Study Guide*.

- Check the answers in the *Study Guide* for the review questions or in the referenced pages of the textbook for the study exercises.

- Reread questions missed on the review test. Answer the questions missed and check answers again.

- If you miss the question a second time, or if you guessed at the answer, return to the referenced pages in the text and review the content.

- After completing the *Study Guide*, you should feel that you have mastery over the material in *Clinical Nursing Skills*.

The authors' intention in writing this *Study Guide* is to assist students to gain experience in answering objective-type questions (the type that are tested on NCLEX), as well as to review the comprehensive content in *Clinical Nursing Skills*. We hope that this workbook will meet students' learning needs.

Sandra F. Smith, RN, MS
Donna Duell, RN, MS

Section I Review Questions

Chapter One
Professional Nursing

QUESTIONS

1. The set of formal guidelines for governing RN's professional action is called
   1. Patient's Bill of Rights.
   2. Nurses' Code of Ethics.
   3. Professional responsibility.
   4. Accountability.

2. As you assume the role of the professional nurse, choose the nursing action that does *not* convey nursing competence.
   1. Dress neatly in appropriate, clean attire.
   2. Speak in slang to help the patient feel comfortable.
   3. Remain professional, not social, when interacting with the patient.
   4. Follow the dress code of the school or facility.

3. Which of the following would NOT be included in a list of skills and functions that professional nurses perform in daily practice (Nurse Practice Act)?
   1. Observe signs and symptoms of illness.
   2. Administer medications according to physician's orders.
   3. Perform diagnostic tests and procedures.
   4. Deliver basic health care services.

4. The best example of the administrative classification of law related to nursing is
   1. Licensure and the State Board of Registered Nursing.
   2. Handling of narcotics.
   3. Patient's rights.
   4. Relationship with employer.

5. Confidential information may NOT be released even by consent of the patient in order to guard against invasion of privacy.
   1. True.
   2. False.

6. Choose the step that is out of sequence when you are preparing for clinical practice.
   1. Read the patient's chart and obtain necessary data for patient care.
   2. Research the patient's diagnosis.
   3. Obtain the clinical assignment in sufficient time to prepare for patient care.
   4. Research the medications the patient is receiving.

7. In medical asepsis, the spread of microorganisms is prevented by the use of _____ and _____ asepsis.
   1. Clean, surgical
   2. Medical, surgical
   3. Sterile, clean
   4. Prevention, medical

ANSWERS

1. CORRECT ANSWER IS 2
The Code of Ethics assists the nurse to problem solve where judgment is required. It encompasses professional responsibility and accountability.
(Pages 2–3)

2. CORRECT ANSWER IS 2
Using slang or inappropriate language does not convey nursing competence as a part of the professional role of the nurse. You should always speak in correct English, use correct grammar and appropriate language.
(Page 3)

3. CORRECT ANSWER IS 3
You would not perform diagnostic tests unless specifically trained to do so.
(Pages 4–5)

4. CORRECT ANSWER IS 1
The other responses refer to tort, constitution, and contract classification respectively.
(Page 7)

5. CORRECT ANSWER IS 2
Confidential information may be released with consent of the patient.
(Page 7)

6. CORRECT ANSWER IS 3
The step out of sequence is number 3. The first step in preparing for clinical practice is to obtain your specific clinical assignment.
(Page 8)

7. CORRECT ANSWER IS 2
While medical asepsis is referred to as "clean technique" and surgical asepsis "sterile technique," these terms are the accepted two forms of asepsis.
(Page 13)

Chapter Two
Nursing Process

QUESTIONS

1. The following steps of the nursing process are listed in proper sequence.

    A. Assessment.
    B. Planning.
    C. Nursing Diagnosis.
    D. Implementation.
    E. Evaluation.
    1. True.
    2. False.

2. The implementation phase of the nursing process is the most important step.

    1. True.
    2. False.

3. Which of the following is the BEST definition of nursing diagnosis?

    1. Nursing diagnosis refers to a health problem or condition that nurses are legally licensed to treat.
    2. Nursing diagnosis includes etiology and relates directly to the defining characteristics.
    3. Nursing diagnosis is the statement of a patient problem derived from the collection of data and its analysis.
    4. Nursing diagnosis is derived from the assessment phase of the nursing process.

4. The nurse gathers assessment data from the following sources:

    A. Patient's history.
    B. Patient's physical assessment.
    C. Laboratory results.
    D. Knowledge of disease process.
    1. A and B only.
    2. B and C only.
    3. B, C, D.
    4. All of the above.

5. The implementation phase of the nursing process is best described as the

    1. Organizational aspects of the nursing process.
    2. Action component of the nursing process.
    3. Foundation for the therapeutic plan of care.
    4. Problem solving foundation of patient care.

Questions 6 and 7 relate to the following situation.

John Jones, a 26-year-old college student, was involved in a motor vehicle accident and sustained a head injury 2 hours before you provide nursing care for him on the surgical nursing unit.

6. The most appropriate goal included in John's care plan should be to monitor

    A. Changes in level of consciousness.
    B. Signs and symptoms.
    C. Intake and output.
    D. Skin color and integrity.

    The phase of the nursing process illustrated in this question is

    1. Assessment.
    2. Planning.
    3. Implementation.
    4. Evaluation.

7. When you are caring for John, the most important nursing action is to

A. Use the Glascow Coma scale every 15 minutes.
B. Select fluids John likes to increase his fluid intake.
C. Position John to increase respiratory effectiveness.
D. Turn John every 2 hours to prevent pressure ulcers.

Which phase of the nursing process is illustrated in this question?

1. Assessment.
2. Planning.
3. Implementation.
4. Evaluation.

8. When a patient is in shock, the most important nursing observation is a/an

A. Increase in pulse rate.
B. Decrease in respirations.
C. Increase in blood pressure.
D. Decrease in blood pressure.

Which phase of the nursing process is illustrated in this question?

1. Assessment.
2. Planning.
3. Implementation.
4. Evaluation.

ANSWERS

1. CORRECT ANSWER IS 2
The proper sequence for the nursing process is assessment, nursing diagnosis, planning, implementation, and evaluation.
(Page 22)

2. CORRECT ANSWER IS 2
All phases are equally important, and while they overlap, each phase must be completed in logical sequence.
(Page 23)

3. CORRECT ANSWER IS 3
All of the other responses are accurate but 3 is the best and most comprehensive definition.
(Page 23)

4. CORRECT ANSWER IS 4
All of the sources listed provide assessment data necessary for developing individualized patient care.
(Page 22)

5. CORRECT ANSWER IS 2
The implementation phase is the action component of the nursing process and involves initiating and completing nursing actions necessary to accomplish identified patient goals.
(Pages 22–23)

6. CORRECT ANSWER IS 2
The planning phase refers to the identification of nursing actions that are strategies to achieve the goals or desired outcomes of nursing care. The answer to the sample question is **A:** Changes in level of consciousness.
(Page 23)

7. CORRECT ANSWER IS 3
The implementation phase refers to the priority nursing actions or interventions performed to accomplish a specified goal. The answer to the sample question is **A:** Use the Glascow Coma scale every 15 minutes.
(Page 23)

8. CORRECT ANSWER IS 1
This is the assessment phase of the nursing process. The answer to the sample question is **A:** Increase in pulse rate.
(Page 23)

Chapter Three
Patient Care Management

QUESTIONS

1. A Patient Care Plan may BEST be described as
   1. Containing the goals and expected outcomes of care.
   2. Providing for quality and consistency of patient care.
   3. Written in several formats, but always including goals and interventions.
   4. Providing a means of staff communication for patient's needs, goals, nursing actions, and discharge criteria.

2. The two types of Patient Care Plans are _____ and _____.
   1. Problem oriented, need oriented
   2. Individualized, standard
   3. Kardex, Rand
   4. Individualized, preprinted

3. Which of the following terms would you expect to find on a standard Patient Care Plan?
   A. Discharge criteria.
   B. Admitting diagnosis.
   C. Unusual problems.
   D. Expected outcome.
   E. Nursing interventions.
   F. Nursing diagnosis.
   1. All except C.
   2. A, B, D, and F.
   3. All except C and F.
   4. B, D, and E.

4. The best explanation for including a checkpoint column in the Patient Care Plan is to
   1. Be sure nurses check each other on their interventions.
   2. Indicate how often the action should be checked, observed, or carried out.
   3. Tell the staff the deadline of when the goal should be met.
   4. Monitor the sequence in which nursing actions should be carried out.

5. Which of the following items would NOT be included in staff (daily) communication process?
   A. Documentation-charting.
   B. Evaluation.
   C. Care conferences.
   D. Patient Care Plans.
   E. Report.
   F. Staff audit.
   1. All except F.
   2. A, C, D, E.
   3. A, B, C, D.
   4. All of the above.

6. The difference between long- and short-term goals is
   1. Long-term goals are designed as stepping stones to meet expected outcomes for each nursing diagnosis.
   2. Long-term goals are updated on a daily basis.
   3. Short-term goals are frequently used interchangeably with discharge criteria.
   4. Short-term goals appear in the form of expected outcomes for each stated problem.

7. The most accurate statement referring to delegating patient care is
   1. Patient care assignments should be based on proximity of rooms to increase effectiveness of nurses' time management.
   2. The patient care plan is the major determinant in identifying the number of hours of patient care needed and, thus, the appropriate staff member for the assignment.
   3. Patient care assignments need to be based on job descriptions of health care workers on the unit.
   4. Determining the number of patients and dividing the assignment equally among all licensed staff members is most important.

8. After all patients are assigned an acuity level, the total patient care acuity number for the nursing unit is used to determine the number of nursing staff required for the shift.
   1. True.
   2. False.

ANSWERS

1. CORRECT ANSWER IS 4
   All of the other responses are correct, but 4 is the most inclusive and comprehensive.
   (Page 30)

2. CORRECT ANSWER IS 2
   The other terms do not refer to types of Patient Care Plans, but to components or format.
   (Page 30)

3. CORRECT ANSWER IS 3
   You would find the terms "usual problems" or "problem/need" stated as a nursing diagnosis, but not the terms themselves.
   (Page 30)

4. CORRECT ANSWER IS 2
   Checkpoint refers to the frequency with which the action or intervention should be checked, observed, or carried out, thus how often it should be charted.
   (Page 34)

5. CORRECT ANSWER IS 2
   Evaluation and staff audit are not a form of communication among the staff.
   (Pages 37–38)

6. CORRECT ANSWER IS 4
   Short-term goals appear in the form of expected outcomes for each problem. Long-term goals are frequently stated as discharge criteria.
   (Page 34)

7. CORRECT ANSWER IS 3
   Job descriptions must be considered when assigning patients to staff members; this ensures that nurses are not working outside their job description and patients receive quality care.
   (Page 37)

8. CORRECT ANSWER IS 1
   The patient acuity level is determined for each shift to adequately plan for staffing needs. For example, the acuity level is determined by 1 PM and used to calculate the number of staff needed for the 3–11 PM shift.
   (Page 38)

Chapter Four
Documentation

QUESTIONS

1. Charting is one of the nurse's most important functions. Which of the following is the most important purpose of charting?
   1. To communicate to other members of the patient's health care team.
   2. To evaluate the staff's performance.
   3. To provide information for a nursing audit.
   4. To enable physicians to monitor nursing care.

2. Complete and accurate charting is essential to protect both the patient and the nurse.
   1. True.
   2. False.

3. Which of the following items would you always include in a patient's chart?
   A. Initial assessment at beginning of shift.
   B. Abnormalities noted during assessment.
   C. Changes in patient's condition.
   D. General verbatim comments.
   E. Patient's response to teaching.
      1. All of the above.
      2. All but D.
      3. All but D and E.
      4. B, C, and E.

4. It is important to record any unscheduled or p.r.n. medication. Would the following be an accurate representation of this type of charting?

   "8 PM. c/o abdominal incisional pain after ambulation. Demerol 50 mg IM for pain."
   1. True.
   2. False.

5. Which of the following statements is the best explanation of source-oriented systems of charting?
   1. This system is based on problems, and the information is charted in chronological order.
   2. It is a common and efficient way of organizing patient information according to the source of information.
   3. This system focuses on the patient's status rather than on the source.
   4. Systematic and well-defined, this method consists of five distinct parts.

6. Which one of the following rules for charting narrative notes does not fit into acceptable charting procedures?
   1. Each entry should be signed with your name and professional status.
   2. Objective facts are more relevant than nursing interpretation.
   3. Behaviors rather than feelings should be charted.
   4. Use of the word "patient" or "pt." is important to designate particular charts.

7. A well-organized POMR system includes progress notes that have a specific format called SOAP. This acronym translates as
   1. Subjective, objective, assessment, and plan.
   2. Summary, objective documentation, assessment, and promoting care.
   3. Symptoms, observations, assessment, and plan.
   4. Subjective, objective, assessment, and priority problems.

8. Computer entries for an individual patient are not part of the permanent record until they are written on the patient's chart.
   1. True.
   2. False.

9. Unusual occurrences (incident reports) serve the purposes of documenting quality of care, identifying areas where in-service education is needed, and recording the details of the incident for legal documentation.

    1. True.
    2. False.

10. When you are charting, it is important to use facts and be specific, not pat phrases, for potential legal problems.

    1. True.
    2. False.

ANSWERS

1. **CORRECT ANSWER IS 1**
   All the answers except 4 are purposes of charting, but 1 is the most inclusive.
   (Page 44)

2. **CORRECT ANSWER IS 1**
   Charting protects both the patient and the nurse from potential legal problems, and charting supports high standards of patient care.
   (Page 44)

3. **CORRECT ANSWER IS 2**
   General verbatim patient comments are not automatically included unless they directly relate to the patient's condition.
   (Page 46)

4. **CORRECT ANSWER IS 1**
   It is important to include patient need, time medication was given, location, dose, and route of administration.
   (Page 46)

5. **CORRECT ANSWER IS 2**
   1 is incorrect because it is not based on problems, but on chronological order. 3 and 4 refer to problem-oriented medical records (POMR).
   (Pages 48–49)

6. **CORRECT ANSWER IS 4**
   The word "patient" should not be used, as the chart belongs to the patient.
   (Page 51)

7. **CORRECT ANSWER IS 1**
   All of the other responses contain at least one distractor.
   (Page 56)

8. **CORRECT ANSWER IS 2**
   Computer entries are part of the patient's permanent record and cannot be deleted.
   (Page 62)

9. **CORRECT ANSWER IS 1**
   These are the three primary purposes for unusual occurrences.
   (Page 63)

10. **CORRECT ANSWER IS 1**
    Facts and specific data are important for legal implications. Pat phrases and global assessments are not appropriate.
    (Page 65)

Chapter Five
Communication and Relationship Skills

QUESTIONS

1. Communication is BEST defined by which of the following statements?

    1. Communication includes both verbal and nonverbal expressions.
    2. Communication is the process of sending and receiving messages.
    3. Communication is a multi-level process between people.
    4. Communication includes messages, gestures, symbols, signs, and words.

2. Gestures, actions, signs, and body movements are examples of _____ communication.

    1. Verbal
    2. Nonverbal
    3. Multi-level
    4. Interaction

3. Reflection, feedback, listening, and open-ended response are examples of

    1. Nursing diagnosis.
    2. Nontherapeutic communication.
    3. Therapeutic communication.
    4. Blocks to communication.

4. Identify the following therapeutic communication technique. "Did you say that you were feeling hot all over?"

    1. Clarification.
    2. Acknowledgment.
    3. Listening.
    4. Neutral response.

5. Which of the following terms would be labeled "blocks to communication"?

    1. Focusing and social response.
    2. False reassurance and giving advice.
    3. Overloading and feedback.
    4. Reflection and invalidation.

6. The best rationale for introducing yourself to a blind patient and telling him exactly what you are doing is that these actions

    1. Illustrate the principle of open communication.
    2. Decrease the patient's anxiety and fear of the unknown.
    3. Are the accepted procedure for beginning a nurse–patient relationship.
    4. Encourage and use clear communication.

7. While silence can be a therapeutic tool, long periods of silence may increase the patient's anxiety level.

    1. True.
    2. False.

8. Relationship can be defined as the interaction between a nurse and a patient with shared therapeutic goals and objectives.

    1. True.
    2. False.

9. Which of the following is NOT a phase in the nurse–patient relationship?

    1. Initiation phase.
    2. Active working phase.
    3. Relationship phase.
    4. Termination phase.

10. It is important to establish trust as a foundation for a nurse–patient relationship.

1. True.
2. False.

11. Anticipate problems of _____ in the beginning of a relationship and plan for their resolution.

1. Facilitating
2. Terminating
3. Charting
4. Initiating

12. The more you say when you are encouraging a patient to describe personal experiences, the more the patient will talk.

1. True.
2. False.

ANSWERS

1. CORRECT ANSWER IS 2
While all of the statements are correct, the most complete definition is 2.
(Page 72)

2. CORRECT ANSWER IS 2
Verbal communication refers to spoken words. 3 and 4 do not apply.
(Page 73)

3. CORRECT ANSWER IS 3
These are all examples of therapeutic, or effective, communication.
(Pages 73–74)

4. CORRECT ANSWER IS 1
Clarifying is checking out or making clear either the intent or meaning of the message.
(Page 73)

5. CORRECT ANSWER IS 2
Both of these techniques are blocks to communication. Focusing (1), feedback (3), and reflection (4) are all therapeutic techniques.
(Pages 75–76)

6. CORRECT ANSWER IS 2
Blind patients become anxious when they hear someone enter the room without talking.
(Page 79)

7. CORRECT ANSWER IS 1
Silence allows the patient to pace and direct his own communication, but long periods of silence may make him uncomfortable.
(Page 73)

8. CORRECT ANSWER IS 1
This is a definition of relationship; characteristics include acceptance, honesty, and empathy.
(Page 76)

9. CORRECT ANSWER IS 3
This is not a specific phase; all phases are components of a relationship.
(Page 77)

10. CORRECT ANSWER IS 1
Trust is the cornerstone of a viable relationship between patient and nurse.
(Page 77)

11. CORRECT ANSWER IS 2
Termination must begin at the initiation of a relationship so problems can be anticipated and resolved.
(Page 77)

12. CORRECT ANSWER IS 2
Minimal verbal activity is important to encourage the patient to talk; therefore, the less you say, the more therapeutic you are when assisting a patient to describe personal experiences.
(Page 79)

Chapter Six
Safe Patient Environment

QUESTIONS

1. The purpose of _____ is to make adjustments that will assist us to control and improve our environment.
   1. Homeostasis
   2. Adaptation
   3. Holism
   4. Surroundings

2. The following terms are dimensions that influence our environment.
   A. Physical dimension = adequate space.
   B. Biological dimension = food and water.
   C. Sociocultural dimension = privacy.
   D. Biological dimension = waste disposal.

   Which of the above dimensions with examples are accurate?
   1. All of the above.
   2. All except C.
   3. A and B.
   4. None of the above.

3. Which of the following would be an appropriate nursing action for preventing mechanical injuries?
   1. Listen to patient's complaints.
   2. Always keep bed in low position.
   3. Make sure floors are free of debris.
   4. Use restraints.

4. The first sign of possible thermal injury for a patient using a hot-water bottle, heating pad, or hot compress is
   1. Tingling sensation in the extremities.
   2. Redness in the area.
   3. Edema.
   4. Pain.

5. Which of the following nursing actions would be inappropriate for a patient using wrist restraints?
   1. Check limbs every 2 hours for circulation.
   2. Change patient's position every 2 hours.
   3. Release restraints every shift.
   4. Put extremities through range of motion every 2 hours.

6. The rationale for fastening wrist restraints under the bed frame and not to the side rail is to prevent injury.
   1. True.
   2. False.

7. Safety belts are applied as follows. Which one is NOT accurate?
   1. For an ambulating patient the belt is fastened around the waist.
   2. For a patient on a gurney the belt is fastened around the abdomen.
   3. For a patient in a wheelchair the belt is fastened around the abdomen and under arm rests.
   4. For a patient on a Stryker frame the belt is fastened around the frame.

8. Charting for applying restraints usually includes which of the following items?

   A. Time and type of restraint.
   B. Rationale for applying restraint.
   C. Physician's orders regarding restraint.
   D. Condition of extremity following application.
   E. Time of removal.
   F. Patient's comments.
   G. Effectiveness of restraint.
   1. All except C and F.
   2. All of the above.
   3. A, B, C, and D.
   4. All except C.

9. The data you would include in nursing charting for applying restraints is the

   1. Physician's orders for restraints.
   2. Patient's statements about the restraints.
   3. Rationale for applying restraints.
   4. Family permission for applying restraints.

ANSWERS

1. CORRECT ANSWER IS 2
Adaptation includes making adjustments in all conscious and unconscious forms.
(Page 86)

2. CORRECT ANSWER IS 1
All of the above dimensions are characteristics that influence the patient's adaptation.
(Pages 89–90)

3. CORRECT ANSWER IS 3
This is a preventive measure. You would not always keep beds in low position or use restraints. Listening to complaints is not always preventive.
(Page 99)

4. CORRECT ANSWER IS 2
Redness, or erythema, is the first sign of possible injury.
(Page 100)

5. CORRECT ANSWER IS 3
It is appropriate to release restraints every 2 hours and administer skin care.
(Page 103)

6. CORRECT ANSWER IS 1
Wrist restraints are tied to the bed frame because side rails are frequently moved up and down.
(Page 103)

7. CORRECT ANSWER IS 4
For a patient on a Stryker frame, the belt is fastened around the patient's abdomen.
(Page 104)

8. CORRECT ANSWER IS 1
Physician orders are already charted and you would only chart patient comments if they were relevant to the patient's condition.
(Page 106)

9. CORRECT ANSWER IS 3
You must include the rationale for applying restraints in the charting. You do not need doctor's orders (they are already on the chart) or family permission. You would chart patient tolerance for restraints, not necessarily what the patient says.
(Page 106)

Chapter Seven
Bathing and Bedmaking

QUESTIONS

1. The most important nursing action in maintaining medical asepsis is
   1. Noncontamination.
   2. Handwashing.
   3. Rinsing hands thoroughly.
   4. Running water.

2. It is necessary to wash your hands for at least 1 minute to remove pathogens.
   1. True.
   2. False.

3. The main purpose for mitering corners of a sheet is to
   1. Secure the bottom sheet.
   2. Make the corner look neat.
   3. Keep bed linens tight.
   4. Follow nursing protocol.

4. The primary difference between a surgical bed and an unoccupied bed is
   1. Linens are fanfolded to side of bed.
   2. Surgical beds include drawsheets.
   3. Unoccupied beds have side rails down on both sides.
   4. Top sheet is pleated to allow for movement of feet.

5. The primary purpose of AM care is to enable the patient to freshen up early in the morning.
   1. True.
   2. False.

6. In performing the skill of bathing, you would begin bathing the patient's face, then his upper body. You would next bathe his
   1. Abdomen.
   2. Upper extremities.
   3. Legs and feet.
   4. Lower extremities.

7. The rationale for using a septi-soft bath for a critically ill patient is that this bath decreases the time it takes to bathe; thus it is less traumatic for the patient.
   1. True.
   2. False.

8. Monitoring the patient's skin condition involves several specific nursing actions. Which of the following does this skill include?
   A. Check skin color.
   B. Assess skin temperature.
   C. Observe for areas of dryness, flaking, and texture.
   D. Examine skin for water retention.
   E. Observe patient for alertness and attention span.
      1. All except D and E.
      2. All of the above.
      3. All except E.
      4. A and B.

9. The best rationale for providing back care to patients in the evening is to promote rest and comfort.
    1. True.
    2. False.

10. The steps of providing evening care for your patient will include
    A. Change dressing, if ordered.
    B. Wash face, hands, and back.
    C. Encourage range-of-motion or active exercises.
    D. Administer sleeping medication, if ordered.
    E. Raise side rails before leaving room.
       1. A, B, C.
       2. All except C.
       3. A, B, D.
       4. All except E.

ANSWERS

1. CORRECT ANSWER IS 2
The most important action to promote medical asepsis is handwashing.
(Page 113)

2. CORRECT ANSWER IS 2
You must wash your hands for at least 30 seconds.
(Page 114)

3. CORRECT ANSWER IS 3
Tight, wrinkle-free sheets help to prevent skin breakdown.
(Page 118)

4. CORRECT ANSWER IS 1
In a surgical bed, linens are fanfolded to the side to facilitate moving surgical patients into the bed.
(Page 119)

5. CORRECT ANSWER IS 1
AM care is provided prior to bathing the patient. This allows the patient to freshen up before breakfast.
(Page 124)

6. CORRECT ANSWER IS 2
It is important to complete washing the upper body before the lower body.
(Page 126)

7. CORRECT ANSWER IS 1
Critically ill patients should not be exposed to the long ordeal of a bath or to changes in temperature for long periods of time.
(Page 128)

8. CORRECT ANSWER IS 3
All of the other actions would be included in monitoring skin condition, and while assessing patient alertness is important, it is not part of the skin assessment.
(Page 132)

9. CORRECT ANSWER IS 1
Back care is an important nursing function for patient comfort.
(Page 136)

10. CORRECT ANSWER IS 2
You will not encourage active exercises or range-of-motion exercises because it is too stimulating at bedtime.
(Page 136)

Chapter Eight
Personal Hygiene

QUESTIONS

1. Which one of the following statements would NOT provide a rationale for providing professional hygienic care?
   1. Level of care influences the patient's perception of the staff.
   2. Professional care increases the patient's confidence in the health care.
   3. Comprehensive care will assist the patient to adapt to the unfamiliar hospital environment.
   4. Hygienic care is a part of the nurse's duty.

2. There are many reasons for providing oral hygiene but the most important is to remove plaque from the oral cavity.
   1. True.
   2. False.

3. You are assigned to provide oral care to an unconscious patient. Considering the following steps of the procedure, which intervention is missing?

   "Gather equipment, wash hands, brush external surfaces, brush inner surfaces of the teeth."
   1. Place bulb syringe or suctioning equipment nearby.
   2. Rinse the mouth cavity.
   3. Floss the teeth.
   4. Check the vital signs.

4. What is the purpose of a shampoo board when you are assigned to shampoo the hair of a patient?
   1. It is used to support patient's head from wheelchair to sink.
   2. It is used to allow soap and water to run off into a basin at the side of the bed.
   3. It is used in place of a basin to collect water.
   4. It is only used when the patient is on a gurney.

5. Patients must have permission to use straight razors, but electric razors are always allowed.
   1. True.
   2. False.

6. The best rationale for cutting toenails straight across is to
   1. Prevent infection.
   2. Prevent trauma to surrounding tissue.
   3. Allow the nurse to clean under nails.
   4. Follow hospital protocol.

7. You are assigned to provide perineal care to a female patient. Which of the following items would be essential to complete this assignment?

   A. Bath blanket.
   B. Bath towels.
   C. Clean surgical gloves.
   D. Cotton balls.
   E. Protective pad.
   F. Drape.
   1. All of the above.
   2. All but F.
   3. All but C and D.
   4. A, B, C, and E.

8. A patient complains of oral mucosal irritation or sensitivity. Which of the following actions are appropriate for this situation?
   1. Keep patient n.p.o. and use Nystatin mouthwash.
   2. Use hydrogen peroxide to loosen and remove debris from mouth.
   3. Rinse mouth with warm water.
   4. Allow patient to drink fluids, but not eat solid foods.

9. To remove lice, the most appropriate nursing actions are

1. Shampoo hair daily for 3 days.
2. Shampoo hair and wash body daily for 1 week.
3. Apply shampoo and leave in place several minutes, repeat in 24 hours if needed.
4. Apply shampoo to hair and lotion to body. Repeat in 24 hours.

10. The appropriate cleansing action for cleaning the eyes is wiping from _____ to _____ canthus.

1. Inner, outer
2. Outer, inner

ANSWERS

1. CORRECT ANSWER IS 4
To perform actions based on duty is not a professional attitude and it will not inspire confidence in the staff.
(Page 144)

2. CORRECT ANSWER IS 2
Removing plaque is a reason, but even more important would be to assess the patient's oral status.
(Page 144)

3. CORRECT ANSWER IS 1
With an unconscious patient, you need to have emergency equipment nearby when you put water in the patient's mouth.
(Page 149)

4. CORRECT ANSWER IS 2
A shampoo board is used only for a patient on bedrest to collect water and soap that runs off into the basin.
(Page 153)

5. CORRECT ANSWER IS 2
Some hospitals do not allow patients to use their own electric razors.
(Page 154)

6. CORRECT ANSWER IS 2
Cutting toenails straight across will prevent trauma as well as ingrown toenails.
(Page 158)

7. CORRECT ANSWER IS 3
Cotton balls and surgical gloves are optional.
(Page 160)

8. CORRECT ANSWER IS 2
The appropriate action is to use hydrogen peroxide. The patient can eat solid food; he need not be n.p.o.
(Page 150)

9. CORRECT ANSWER IS 3
Head lice requires shampoo and body lice requires soap followed by lotion application. The procedure should be repeated in 24 hours if needed.
(Page 155)

10. CORRECT ANSWER IS 1
Cleansing the eye from the inner to the outer canthus prevents particles and fluid from entering the nasolacrimal duct.
(Page 163)

Chapter Nine
Vital Signs

QUESTIONS

1. The main purpose for obtaining vital signs on a patient is to
   1. Determine the patient's regulatory mechanisms.
   2. Obtain a total picture of the patient's health status.
   3. Provide information to determine the patient's homeostatic balance.
   4. Determine variation in temperature, pulse, and respiration.

2. The _____ is the critical temperature level to which the regulatory mechanisms attempt to maintain the body's core temperature.
   1. Body core
   2. Body thermostat
   3. Set point
   4. Hypothermic level

3. Which of the following terms does NOT describe a characteristic of the pulse wave (the forceful ejection of blood through the artery)?
   1. Blood viscosity.
   2. Elasticity of larger vessels.
   3. Capillary resistance.
   4. Number of beats/minute.

4. Normal respiratory rate for a resting adult is 12–18 breaths/minute.
   1. True.
   2. False.

5. Choose the major factors that affect blood pressure.
   A. Cardiac output.
   B. Peripheral vascular resistance.
   C. Blood volume.
   D. Blood viscosity.
   E. Systolic and diastolic levels.
   F. Hormones and enzymes.
   1. All of the above.
   2. All but E.
   3. All but E and F.
   4. Only A and B.

6. Korotkoff sounds are
   1. Phases of systolic and diastolic pressure readings.
   2. The same as systolic and diastolic readings.
   3. Variations of pressure readings.
   4. The normal blood pressure reading.

7. The _____ artery is most commonly used for taking a pulse.
   1. Apical
   2. Peripheral
   3. Radial
   4. Apical-radial

8. You are taking a peripheral pulse that is very weak. You should press down firmly to palpate a weak pulse.
   1. True.
   2. False.

9. You are assessing your patient's breathing pattern and you determine that he is having Cheyne-Stokes respirations because

   1. Periods of hyperpnea alternate with periods of apnea.
   2. Periods of tachypnea alternate with periods of apnea.
   3. Both rate and depth of respirations have increased.
   4. The patient has deep, regular, sighing respirations.

10. You are assigned to take Mr. Marvin's blood pressure. Which of the following actions is incorrect?

    1. Wrap cuff snugly around upper arm.
    2. Palpate brachial artery before placing diaphragm on arm.
    3. Open valve on manometer pump.
    4. Inflate cuff 30 mm Hg above level at which pulsations are no longer heard.

11. Flush pressures are taken on small infants or adults when you cannot auscultate or palpate blood pressure readings.

    1. True.
    2. False.

12. The best definition for pulse deficit is

    1. Rhythm is regular but amplitude alternates beat to beat.
    2. Pulse diminishes in amplitude with inspiration, and stroke volume is decreased.
    3. Heart rate counted at apex is greater than rate at radial pulse.
    4. Pulse occurs with premature beats and there is a disturbance in rhythm.

ANSWERS

1. CORRECT ANSWER IS 2
   The major objective is to obtain a total picture of a patient's health status. It will also yield important baseline information for future assessments.
   (Page 170)

2. CORRECT ANSWER IS 3
   Set point refers to the level at which the body attempts to maintain core temperature.
   (Page 171)

3. CORRECT ANSWER IS 4
   The pulse is an index of the heart's rate and rhythm, but the force of the wave is not influenced by beats/minute.
   (Page 173)

4. CORRECT ANSWER IS 1
   Normal rate for a resting adult is 12–18 breaths/minute. Infant rate is 24–30.
   (Page 174)

5. CORRECT ANSWER IS 2
   Systolic and diastolic pressure provide information about the condition of the heart, arteries, and arterioles. The remaining terms affect the pressure.
   (Page 175)

6. CORRECT ANSWER IS 1
   These sounds or phases begin at the first systolic reading and end at the last sound.
   (Page 176)

7. CORRECT ANSWER IS 3
   The radial artery is most commonly used, as it is easily accessible. Apical pulse is taken for irregular rhythms or for patients receiving heart medications.
   (Page 183)

8. CORRECT ANSWER IS 2
   You will obliterate a weak pulse with too much pressure. Palpate weak pulses very gently.
   (Page 187)

9. CORRECT ANSWER IS 1
Hyperpnea is followed by periods of apnea.
(Page 191)

10. CORRECT ANSWER IS 3
You close, not open, the valve on the manometer pump.
(Page 193)

11. CORRECT ANSWER IS 1
Flush pressures are not taken routinely. The reading is between systolic and diastolic, and it is not as accurate.
(Page 196)

12. CORRECT ANSWER IS 3
The other definitions are respectively: pulsus alterans, pulsus paradoxus, and bigeminal pulse.
(Page 199)

Chapter Ten
Body Mechanics and Positioning

QUESTIONS

1. The musculoskeletal system is made up of

   1. Skeletal muscles.
   2. Joints.
   3. Bones.
   4. Tissue.

   Which of the above terms does NOT fit?

2. The primary rationale for the nurse to use proper body mechanics is to

   1. Protect the patient.
   2. Prevent injuries.
   3. Establish body alignment.
   4. Maintain body alignment.

3. When working at a low surface level, you should not stoop or bend over to implement proper body mechanics.

   1. True.
   2. False.

4. When placing the patient in semi-Fowler's position, the head of the bed will be at a _____ angle.

   1. 45-degree
   2. 30-degree
   3. 60-degree
   4. Slanted

5. To perform the skill "turning to the side-lying position," you would lower the head of the bed, elevate bed to working height, move patient to your side of the bed, and flex patient's knees. The next intervention would be

   1. Roll the patient on his side.
   2. Reposition patient.
   3. Place one hand on patient's hip and other on shoulder.
   4. Position patient's arms so they are not under his body.

6. When moving the patient up in bed, remove the pillow and place it at the head of the bed. The rationale for this action is to

   1. Get it out of the way.
   2. Prevent the patient from striking his head.
   3. Facilitate completing the procedure.
   4. Enable the patient to push from his knees.

7. You are assigned to move the patient from the bed to a chair. What is the first appropriate intervention?

   1. Dangle the patient at his bedside.
   2. Put nonslip shoes or slippers on patient's feet.
   3. Rock the patient and pivot.
   4. Position patient so that he is comfortable.

8. Which type of patient would not be appropriate to move with a Hoyer lift?

   1. CVA.
   2. Immobilized.
   3. Obese.
   4. Back injured.

23

9. Your team is assigned to log-roll Mr. Johnson. The appropriate position for staff members is
   1. One nurse at patient's head and the second nurse at patient's shoulder and hip.
   2. Two nurses at patient's head (one on either side) and the third nurse at patient's hip.
   3. One nurse at patient's head, second nurse at shoulder, and third nurse at hip—all on the same side of the patient.
   4. One nurse at patient's head, second nurse at patient's shoulder and hip, and third nurse on opposite side to hold drawsheet and support torso.

10. The primary purpose of using a footboard is to
    1. Encourage flexion.
    2. Prevent plantar flexion.
    3. Ensure proper positioning.
    4. Prevent thrombophlebitis.

ANSWERS

1. CORRECT ANSWER IS 4
Tissue covers and cushions the ends of the bones but is not a major structure of this system.
(Page 202)

2. CORRECT ANSWER IS 2
Good body mechanics preserve the nurse's own musculoskeletal system from injury.
(Page 203)

3. CORRECT ANSWER IS 1
Stooping may harm your back so it is important to flex the knees and use thigh and gluteal muscles to do the work.
(Page 205)

4. CORRECT ANSWER IS 2
Semi-Fowler's position is a 30-degree angle of the head of the bed.
(Page 209)

5. CORRECT ANSWER IS 3
Before rolling patient on his side, your hands must be in the correct position to turn. 4 would be the final intervention.
(Page 210)

6. CORRECT ANSWER IS 2
With no cushion, the patient may hit his head as you move him up in bed.
(Page 211)

7. CORRECT ANSWER IS 1
Before moving the patient, dangling is important to stabilize patient and assess that he won't become dizzy from a drop in blood pressure.
(Page 213)

8. CORRECT ANSWER IS 4
You would not use a Hoyer lift for a patient with spinal cord (back) injury.
(Page 215)

9. CORRECT ANSWER IS 4
To correctly logroll a patient, three nurses must work together to maintain body alignment: two on one side and the third nurse on the opposite side to support the patient.
(Page 216)

10. CORRECT ANSWER IS 2
The main purpose of a footboard is to prevent footdrop or plantar flexion. Answer 3 is not incorrect, but it is too general.
(Page 216)

Chapter Eleven
Exercise and Ambulation

QUESTIONS

1. All joints should be put through full range of motion once a day for 20 minutes.
   1. True.
   2. False.

2. Passive exercises are helpful in maintaining muscle mass.
   1. True.
   2. False.

3. When monitoring continuous passive motion, the machine will be kept on the patient for _____ hours per day.
   1. 2–3
   2. 12–14
   3. 4–6
   4. 24

4. When ambulating a patient with a CVA (cerebral vascular accident) the nurse should stand on the affected side for support.
   1. True.
   2. False.

5. Your instructions to a patient using a four-point crutch walking gait include moving the
   1. Right foot, then the right crutch.
   2. Right crutch, then the right foot.
   3. Right crutch, then the left foot.
   4. Left foot, then the left crutch.

6. Your initial instruction to a patient on the use of crutches to move upstairs should be
   1. Start with crutches and unaffected leg on the same level.
   2. Start with crutches and affected leg on same level.
   3. Place crutches on the step after affected leg is moved up the stair.
   4. Place crutches on the stair and then move the affected leg to the stair.

7. Abduction is defined as the movement of a bone toward the midline of the body.
   1. True.
   2. False.

8. Match the definition in Column B with the appropriate joint movement in Column A.

Column A	Column B
___ 1. Protraction	A. Movement of a bone around its own axis.
___ 2. Pronation	B. Rotation of body so face and abdomen are downward.
___ 3. Eversion	C. Movement of clavicle or mandible forward on a plane parallel to the ground.
___ 4. Retraction	D. Movement of clavicle or mandible backward on a plane parallel to the ground.
___ 5. Rotation	E. Turning outward.
	F. Turning inward.

9. Bones serve as levers and joints serve as fulcrums of these levers.
   1. True.
   2. False.

10. A muscle that moves a body part usually extends over that part.
    1. True.
    2. False.

11. Continuous passive motion machines (CPM) are set to cycle _____ times each minute.
    1. 1–3
    2. 4–6
    3. 3–8
    4. 2–10

12. You are assigned to teach a patient about ambulating with a cane. You instruct the patient to
    1. Place the cane 12 inches in front and slightly to the side of the foot.
    2. First move the affected leg forward and then the unaffected leg.
    3. Ambulate only with another person standing on the unaffected side.
    4. Hold the cane close to the body for better support before ambulating.

ANSWERS

1. CORRECT ANSWER IS 2
   All joints should be put through five full range of motion exercises twice a day.
   (Page 227)

2. CORRECT ANSWER IS 2
   Passive exercises only help prevent contractures; they do not maintain muscle mass.
   (Page 227)

3. CORRECT ANSWER IS 2
   The continuous passive motion machine is kept on the patient for 12–14 hours every day.
   (Page 230)

4. CORRECT ANSWER IS 2
   For best support the nurse should stand on the unaffected side of a patient with a CVA.
   (Page 233)

5. CORRECT ANSWER IS 3
   The crutch is always moved first, and then the foot on the opposite side is moved forward.
   (Page 238)

6. CORRECT ANSWER IS 1
   The crutches and unaffected leg start on the same level; then, the unaffected leg is moved to the step followed by the crutches and affected leg.
   (Page 240)

7. CORRECT ANSWER IS 2
   This definition refers to adduction. In abduction the movement is away from the midline of the body.
   (Page 242)

8. The correct answers: 1=C, 2=B, 3=E, 4=D, 5=A.
   (Page 223)

9. CORRECT ANSWER IS 1
   Muscle function is produced by pulling on bones, as bones serve as levers. Joints serve as fulcrums of these levers.
   (Page 223)

10. CORRECT ANSWER IS 2
    Muscles that move a body part do not extend over than part.
    (Page 223)

11. CORRECT ANSWER IS 4
The number of cycles is dependent on the patient's condition and will be ordered by the physician. The range is 2–10 cycles/minute.
(Page 230)

12. CORRECT ANSWER IS 1
This position provides the best balance because the center of gravity is within the base of support.
(Page 235)

Chapter Twelve
Admission and Discharge

QUESTIONS

1. Which of the following statements relating to the admission of a patient is false?
   1. Assessment is the first nursing action that occurs when a new patient is admitted to a unit.
   2. It is important to assess all aspects of the patient—his physical, emotional, and intellectual status.
   3. A primary objective is to assist the patient to adapt to the hospital environment.
   4. The admitting procedure is important because it assists the patient to adapt as well as establishes a data base of information.

2. When a patient has been transferred to your unit, you would expect a report from the transferring nurse based on both the Patient Care Plan and the Kardex.
   1. True.
   2. False.

3. Weighing the patient is a specific procedure. Which nursing action does NOT belong?
   1. Weigh the patient at the same time every day, usually in the evening.
   2. Always have the patient void before weighing.
   3. Use the same scale each time you weigh.
   4. Check that the patient wears the same type of clothing every time he is weighed.

4. In the question above, one statement relates to using the same scale each time you weigh the patient. The rationale for this action is
   1. The patient becomes familiar with one particular method.
   2. You know that the scale will be balanced correctly.
   3. The same scale gives consistency in weight from day to day.
   4. The physician orders a particular scale and the nurse must follow orders.

5. The reason that patients are discharged in a wheelchair is for
   1. Comfort.
   2. Convenience.
   3. Safety.
   4. Rehabilitation.

6. Your patient insists on being discharged from the hospital against medical advice. From a legal standpoint, what is the most important nursing action?
   1. Notify the supervisor and hospital administration.
   2. Ascertain exactly why the patient wants to leave.
   3. Put all appropriate forms in the patient's chart before he leaves the hospital.
   4. Request that the patient sign the AMA form.

29

ANSWERS

1. CORRECT ANSWER IS 1
The first nursing action should be to introduce yourself to the patient. This occurs before any assessment actions.
(Page 248)

2. CORRECT ANSWER IS 1
Both Patient Care Plan and Kardex are important tools to transmit information.
(Page 252)

3. CORRECT ANSWER IS 1
The patient should be weighed in the morning before breakfast.
(Page 253)

4. CORRECT ANSWER IS 3
The same scale gives consistency and eliminates as many variables as possible.
(Page 253)

5. CORRECT ANSWER IS 3
Transportation by wheelchair can prevent falls and injury.
(Page 255)

6. CORRECT ANSWER IS 4
All of the above actions would be appropriate to carry out. Legally, signing the AMA form is most important.
(Page 257)

Chapter Thirteen
Basic Physical Assessment

QUESTIONS

1. Decorticate posturing is the result of brainstem lesions.
   1. True.
   2. False.

2. When performing a pupil assessment, you should move the pen light from the inner canthus (near nose) to the outside to observe the reaction to light.
   1. True.
   2. False.

3. Reflexes assessed for adult patients include all of the following except
   A. Blink.
   B. Grasp.
   C. Gag.
   D. Deep tendon.
      1. A and C.
      2. B.
      3. D.
      4. A.

4. The face and trunk are the areas where jaundice is most frequently observed.
   1. True.
   2. False.

5. Petechiae are examples of macules.
   1. True.
   2. False.

6. The patient has an injury to the seventh cranial nerve. Your assessment will identify an abnormality in
   1. Closing the eyelid.
   2. Trapezius muscle movement.
   3. Hearing.
   4. Tongue control.

7. Conjunctivitis results in a greenish discharge from the eye.
   1. True.
   2. False.

8. Battle's sign is an indication of a perforated tympanic membrane.
   1. True.
   2. False.

9. When auscultating the lung fields, you will start at the base of the lungs and move toward the apex.
   1. True.
   2. False.

10. Bronchovesicular breath sounds are heard normally over the
    1. Lung base.
    2. Trachea above the sternal notch.
    3. Mainstem bronchi below the clavicle.
    4. Entire lung parenchyma.

11. An S_2 heart sound represents
    1. Closure of the aortic valve.
    2. Closure of the mitral valve.
    3. An atrial gallop.
    4. A ventricular gallop.

31

12. The tricuspid valve sound is best heard at the

1. Second intercostal space, left sternal border.
2. Second intercostal space at the sternal border.
3. Midclavicular line, fifth intercostal space.
4. Left, fifth intercostal space at sternal border.

13. Increased or hyperactive bowel sounds can result from a partial bowel obstruction.

1. True.
2. False.

14. In assessing the mental status of a patient, the factors most likely to be observed are

A. Physical appearance.
B. Motor activity.
C. Perceptions.
D. Skin condition.
  1. B and C.
  2. A and C.
  3. All except D.
  4. All of the above.

ANSWERS

1. CORRECT ANSWER IS 2
Decorticate posturing is a result of a lesion on the corticospinal tract near the cerebral hemisphere.
(Page 264)

2. CORRECT ANSWER IS 2
The penlight is moved toward the patient's eye from the side position.
(Page 264)

3. CORRECT ANSWER IS 2
The grasp reflex is assessed in newborns only.
(Page 266)

4. CORRECT ANSWER IS 1
Jaundice is best observed under natural light around the face and trunk.
(Page 269)

5. CORRECT ANSWER IS 1
There is not an elevation on the skin with macules. A first degree burn is also an example of macules.
(Page 270)

6. CORRECT ANSWER IS 1
The seventh cranial nerve supplies both motor and sensory function. The eyelid closure is a result of the motor function.
(Page 272)

7. CORRECT ANSWER IS 2
The discharge is a thick white color when conjunctivitis occurs.
(Page 273)

8. CORRECT ANSWER IS 2
Battle's sign, ecchymosis behind the ear, is a sign of a basilar skull fracture.
(Page 274)

9. CORRECT ANSWER IS 2
Auscultation begins at the apex and moves bilaterally toward the base of the lungs.
(Page 275)

10. CORRECT ANSWER IS 3
These sounds are hollow, muffled sounds that are heard over the bronchial area.
(Page 279)

11. CORRECT ANSWER IS 1
The S_2 heart sound represents closure of the aortic and pulmonic valves.
(Page 280)

12. CORRECT ANSWER IS 4
The tricuspid valve separates the right atrium and ventricle; therefore, it is heard best at the sternal border, fifth intercostal space.
(Page 280)

13. CORRECT ANSWER IS 1
The sound is high-pitched and tinkling or comes in "rushes" followed by silence as obstruction progresses.
(Page 283)

14. CORRECT ANSWER IS 3
Skin condition is not usually assessed during the mental assessment. The cleanliness of the patient is frequently observed but not the presence of lesions, and so on.
(Pages 286–287)

Chapter Fourteen
Infection Control and AIDS Care

QUESTIONS

1. The most important method of preventing the spread of infection is through
   1. The use of a mask.
   2. Handwashing.
   3. Gowning and gloving.
   4. Appropriate disposal of soiled equipment.

2. Handwashing should take _____ seconds and is completed by keeping the fingers pointed _____.
   1. 30, upward
   2. 30, downward
   3. 60, upward
   4. 60, downward

3. Place in sequence the steps for leaving an isolation room. (The steps may be used more than once.)
   A. Wash your hands.
   B. Take off mask.
   C. Take off gown.
   D. Take off gloves.
      1. D, B, C, A.
      2. D, A, B, A, C.
      3. D, C, B, A.
      4. D, B, A, C.

4. Patients cannot be transported out of their room without contaminating the surroundings.
   1. True.
   2. False.

5. Disposal precautions are followed for
   1. Isolation equipment.
   2. Syringes and needles.
   3. Thermometers.
   4. Plastic items.

6. AIDS is contagious through all of the following mechanisms EXCEPT
   1. Transfused blood products.
   2. Intravenous drug use with shared needles.
   3. Body-to-body contact.
   4. Broken skin area.

7. In which situation would gloves not be necessary?
   1. When in contact with urine.
   2. When suctioning patients.
   3. Changing an ostomy pouch.
   4. Delivering a food tray to an AIDS patient.

8. Protective eyewear should be worn at all times when
   1. Giving personal care to an AIDS patient.
   2. Bathing a neonate for the first time.
   3. Drawing cord blood.
   4. Taking specimens to the lab.

9. When an area becomes inflamed, _____ is/are released, creating increased vascular permeability around the injured site.

   1. Plasmin
   2. Histamine
   3. Kinen
   4. Leukocytes

10. Two major factors that determine whether an infection occurs include

    1. Age and general health status.
    2. Underlying disease status and exposure time to infectious agent.
    3. Inherent health and immunologic status.
    4. Type of organism and age.

ANSWERS

1. CORRECT ANSWER IS 2
   Handwashing is the single most important method of preventing the spread of infection.
   (Page 303)

2. CORRECT ANSWER IS 2
   Keep fingers pointed downward to facilitate removal of organisms.
   (Page 303)

3. CORRECT ANSWER IS 3
   This protocol prevents contamination of the nurse by isolation clothing.
   (Page 306)

4. CORRECT ANSWER IS 2
   Patients can be transported out of their room by donning specific clothing necessary to prevent the spread of disease.
   (Page 308)

5. CORRECT ANSWER IS 2
   Equipment, thermometers, and plastic items are disinfected or sterilized. Syringes and needles must be handled with disposal precautions.
   (Page 308)

6. CORRECT ANSWER IS 3
   Research indicates that there must be a break in the skin or mucous membranes and blood-to blood or body fluid contact for transmission to occur.
   (Page 299)

7. CORRECT ANSWER IS 4
   The first three situations could result in transmission of the HIV virus.
   (Page 300)

8. CORRECT ANSWER IS 3
   Blood could accidentally splash on the skin or mucous membrane of the nurse.
   (Page 300)

9. CORRECT ANSWER IS 2
   Histamine release leads to the release of chemotoxic agents, which summon phagocytes into the vascular and tissue spaces.
   (Page 292)

10. CORRECT ANSWER IS 3
    In addition to inherent health and immunological status, virulence and number of organisms, exposure time and attachment of the organism to the susceptible site play a major role in determining whether an infection will occur.
    (Page 293)

Chapter Fifteen
Medication Administration

1. Before clinical practice, it is imperative to research unfamiliar drugs.
    1. True.
    2. False.

2. When checking medication cards against the Kardex, check the medication listed on the Kardex and then select the appropriate card.
    1. True.
    2. False.

3. A medication order states that you are to give one fluid dram of the liquid. You have a medication cup which is measured in mLs. How many mLs will you administer?
    1. 1 mL.
    2. 4 mL.
    3. 8 mL.
    4. 30 mL.

4. Unit dose medications taken from the drug cart should be checked and placed unwrapped in a medication cup before taking to the patient's room.
    1. True.
    2. False.

5. Medications should be documented in the chart just before administering them to the patient.
    1. True.
    2. False.

6. The medication cart is taken to the patient's room when using the unit dose system.
    1. True.
    2. False

7. Safety checks that should be carried out when administering medications include
    A. Asking the patient to state his name.
    B. Checking the room number.
    C. Calling the patient by name.
    D. Checking the identaband.
    1. D only.
    2. C, D.
    3. A, C, D.
    4. All of the above.

8. Narcotics are checked every 24 hours by the charge nurse.
    1. True.
    2. False.

9. When a patient experiences a severe anaphylactic reaction to a medication, your initial response would be to
    1. Start an IV.
    2. Assess vital signs.
    3. Place the patient in a supine position.
    4. Prepare equipment for intubation.

10. Sublingual medications are not administered to unconscious patients.
    1. True.
    2. False.

11. The most appropriate needle used for administering an intramuscular injection into the deltoid muscle is a
    1. 25 gauge, 5/8" needle.
    2. 22 gauge, 1" needle.
    3. 22 gauge, 1 1/2" needle.
    4. 25 gauge, 1 1/2 " needle.

12. When withdrawing medications from an ampule, the first step is to inject air into the ampule and then withdraw the medication.

    1. True.
    2. False.

13. The needle is inserted at a 20- to 30-degree angle when administering an intradermal injection.

    1. True.
    2. False.

14. Place in sequence the steps for administering a subcutaneous injection.

    A. Express air bubbles from syringe.
    B. Chart medication.
    C. Cleanse area with an alcohol wipe.
    D. Take off needle guard.
       1. B, A, D, C.
       2. A, D, C, B.
       3. C, D, A, B.
       4. D, A, C, B.

15. When administering two types of insulin, you withdraw the long acting insulin into the syringe before the short acting insulin.

    1. True.
    2. False.

16. A major advantage of using an insulin pump is that the patient does not have to adjust life and eating habits to coincide with insulin action time.

    1. True.
    2. False.

17. When administering an IM injection, you pull back on the plunger and blood returns. Your initial action is to

    1. Continue to inject the medication.
    2. Reposition needle slightly and inject the medication.
    3. Remove needle and inject into new area.
    4. Withdraw needle and prepare a new injection.

18. All of the following actions are carried out when administering a medication using the Z-track method except

    1. Placing 0.3 to 0.5 mL of air into the syringe.
    2. Using a 3-inch needle.
    3. Inserting the needle and injecting medication without aspirating.
    4. Pulling skin laterally away from injection site before inserting needle.

19. The correct action for instilling eye drops is to instill drops

    1. At the outer canthus of the eye.
    2. Over the conjunctiva.
    3. Directly on the cornea.
    4. Into the center of the conjunctival sac.

20. Ear medications for adults are instilled by

    1. Lifting the pinna upward and backward.
    2. Pulling the auricle downward and backward.
    3. Lifting the auricle upward and backward.
    4. Lifting the pinna downward and backward.

ANSWERS

1. CORRECT ANSWER IS 1
   In order to safely administer drugs to patients, all unfamiliar drugs should be researched.
   (Page 323)

2. CORRECT ANSWER IS 1
   This method of checking medications should prevent errors in omission due to lost cards.
   (Page 323)

3. CORRECT ANSWER IS 2
   4 mL is equal to one dram.
   (Page 324)

4. CORRECT ANSWER IS 2
   The medication wrapper should not be removed until the medication is dispensed to the patient. This allows an additional safety check for correct medication and dosage.
   (Page 324)

5. **CORRECT ANSWER IS 2**
Medications are documented immediately following administration to the patient.
(Page 325)

6. **CORRECT ANSWER IS 1**
Carts are taken from room to room when using the unit dose system.
(Page 327)

7. **CORRECT ANSWER IS 4**
All of the actions are carried out to prevent medication errors.
(Page 327)

8. **CORRECT ANSWER IS 2**
Narcotics are checked every 8 hours by an oncoming and off-going nurse.
(Page 327)

9. **CORRECT ANSWER IS 3**
The shock position is necessary to maintain vital signs. The other interventions may be carried out but are not initial actions.
(Page 331)

10. **CORRECT ANSWER IS 2**
Sublingual medications can be administered to comatose patients.
(Page 332)

11. **CORRECT ANSWER IS 1**
A 23 or 25 gauge 5/8" needle is the most appropriate size when using the deltoid muscle.
(Page 334)

12. **CORRECT ANSWER IS 2**
Air is not injected into an ampule as it causes displacement of the medication.
(Page 335)

13. **CORRECT ANSWER IS 2**
The needle is inserted at a 10- to 15-degree angle when administering an intradermal injection.
(Page 338)

14. **CORRECT ANSWER IS 3**
The injection area is cleansed before manipulating the syringe and charting the medication.
(Page 338)

15. **CORRECT ANSWER IS 2**
Short acting insulin is withdrawn first to prevent possible contamination of the short acting insulin bottle by the longer acting insulin.
(Pages 340, 342)

16. **CORRECT ANSWER IS 1**
The insulin pump gives lifestyle advantages and schedule flexibility for the patient.
(Page 342)

17. **CORRECT ANSWER IS 4**
In terms of safety and asepsis, this answer is correct. However, in actual practice, the needle is often repositioned by pulling back slightly.
(Page 345)

18. **CORRECT ANSWER IS 3**
Pulling back on the plunger, or aspirating, will ensure that you have not entered a blood vessel.
(Page 347)

19. **CORRECT ANSWER IS 4**
Drops instilled in the center of the sac will assist in distributing the medication over the entire surface of the conjunctiva and anterior eyeball.
(Page 353)

20. **CORRECT ANSWER IS 1**
This maneuver will straighten out the ear canal to ensure that medication reaches the appropriate area.
(Page 356)

Chapter Sixteen
Pain Management

QUESTIONS

1. The most important information gathered while completing an assessment of pain in an adult client is

    1. Observation of body language.
    2. Verbal report from patient.
    3. Palpation of painful areas.
    4. Nonverbal responses from patient.

2. The pain experience is mainly considered to be what type of sensation?

    1. Physical.
    2. Physiological.
    3. Psychosocial.
    4. Mixture of all of the above.

3. TENS (transcutaneous electric nerve stimulation) is thought to relieve pain by any one of the following responses EXCEPT

    1. Increased endorphin production.
    2. Fatigue of peripheral nerve fibers.
    3. Stimulation of efferent nerve fibers.
    4. Blockade of primary afferent fibers.

4. The third phase in biofeedback establishes a link between internal sensations and the effect on a body system.

    1. True.
    2. False.

5. Your instructions to a patient using relaxation techniques for pain control should include the following information after telling him to breathe in and out slowly.

    1. Inhale deeply and hold your breath.
    2. Tense the painful area.
    3. Completely relax the painful area.
    4. Find a point of tension in your body.

6. PCA Infuser Pumps enable the patient to control three parameters of medication delivery. Which parameter is not controlled by the patient?

    1. Stopping and starting the infusion.
    2. Administering a bolus dose.
    3. Titrating the hourly dose within a preset range.
    4. Deciding on dose parameters.

7. Pain is controlled by setting the PCA (patient-controlled IV analgesia) pump's hourly infusion rate to equal no more than 20 mL/hour.

    1. True.
    2. False.

8. It is important to let patients know that PCA will allow them to control their pain level, allowing them to feel less helpless.

    1. True.
    2. False.

ANSWERS

1. CORRECT ANSWER IS 2
The patient's verbal input concerning his pain is the most important information. Pain is totally subjective and only the patient can explain his pain experience.
(Page 368)

2. CORRECT ANSWER IS 4
All three sensations—physical, physiological, and psychosocial—play a role in the pain experience.
(Page 368)

3. CORRECT ANSWER IS 3
Stimulation of afferent, not efferent, nerve fibers is a theory generated as to the function of TENS. Increased endorphin production and fatigue of peripheral nerve fibers play a role in the function of TENS.
(Page 372)

4. CORRECT ANSWER IS 1
This statement is true. The sensation may be felt as warmth around the heart and the effect is slowing heart rate.
(Page 373)

5. CORRECT ANSWER IS 4
After asking a patient to find a point of tension in the body, have him tense the muscles in the area.
(Page 375)

6. CORRECT ANSWER IS 4
The patient may control all the listed parameters except the dose, which is set by the physician.
(Page 380)

7. CORRECT ANSWER IS 1
The pump's hourly infusion rate is set to equal the total mg/hour needed to control pain. The maximum is 20 mL/hour.
(Page 381)

8. CORRECT ANSWER IS 1
When patients know they control their pain level, they feel less helpless.
(Page 385)

Chapter Seventeen
Nutritional Management

QUESTIONS

1. When analyzing a basic nutritional assessment, all of the following factors are essential and should be considered except
   1. Food preference.
   2. Meal patterns.
   3. Sociocultural factors.
   4. Elimination schedule.

2. Feeding a patient should encompass all activities except
   1. Asking the order in which he wants the food to be fed to him.
   2. Alternating foods.
   3. Having all food and fluids handled only by the nurse.
   4. Talking with the patient during the meal.

3. A patient with advanced cirrhosis of the liver will most likely be placed on a _____ diet.
   1. High protein, low potassium
   2. Low protein and sodium
   3. Fat controlled, low potassium and sodium
   4. High protein and fat, low carbohydrate

4. A patient with renal disease will most likely be placed on a _____ diet.
   1. High protein, high carbohydrate, and low potassium
   2. High protein, high fat, and low carbohydrate
   3. Low calcium, low sodium, and high purine
   4. Low protein, potassium, and sodium

5. Foods rich in fat-soluble vitamins include
   A. Citrus foods.
   B. Lean meat.
   C. Whole milk.
   D. Yellow vegetables.
   1. A, B.
   2. C, D.
   3. A, C, D.
   4. All except D.

6. When instructing a patient to follow a low potassium diet, you will tell him to avoid which of the following foods?
   A. Fish.
   B. Raw apples.
   C. Dry cereal.
   D. French bread.
   1. A only.
   2. B, D.
   3. A, B.
   4. All except A.

7. Which one of the following statements is true concerning a postoperative diet?
   1. A patient undergoing major surgery can usually have a soft diet the night before surgery.
   2. Approximately 2800 calories are required daily for tissue repair.
   3. Daily fluid intake should be 1500 mL for an uncomplicated surgical procedure.
   4. A mechanical, soft diet should be given the second postoperative day.

8. A nasogastric tube is measured from the _____ to the _____ and to the _____ before insertion.

   1. Tip of the nose, chin, middle of sternum
   2. Tip of the ear lobe, chin, xiphoid process
   3. Tip of the ear, bridge of the nose, xiphoid process
   4. Tip of the nose, tip of the ear lobe, xiphoid process

9. Considering the following methods, the best one for checking nasogastric tube placement is to

   1. Ensure that tube is inserted to black line nearest measured point.
   2. Inject 10 mL normal saline and listen for whooshing sound.
   3. Listen for rush of air using stethoscope over stomach while injecting air through nasogastric tube.
   4. Observe for choking sounds after nasogastric tube is inserted.

10. Irrigating a nasogastric tube should be carried out using which one of the following protocols?

    1. Gently instill 20 mL normal saline and then withdraw solution.
    2. Instill 30 mL sterile water and then withdraw solution.
    3. Instill 30 mL sterile saline, forcefully if necessary, and allow fluid to flow into basin for return.
    4. Gently instill 20 mL sterile saline and then allow fluid to flow into basin for return.

11. You are administering a nasogastric feeding. While aspirating the stomach contents, you obtain 50 mL of residual. Your next action is to

    1. Discard aspirate and begin tube feeding.
    2. Replace aspirate and begin tube feeding.
    3. Discard aspirate and hold the tube feeding.
    4. Replace aspirate and hold the tube feeding.

12. You are assigned to a patient with a central vein IV infusing hyperalimentation solution. Nursing care for the shift will most likely include

    1. Preparing the solution prior to use.
    2. Maintaining the correct amount of solution administered hourly by adjusting the flow rate.
    3. Checking urine specific gravity, sugar, and acetone every 4 hours.
    4. Changing the IV filter and tubing with each bottle change.

13. Side effects of IV lipid infusions include

    A. Flushing.
    B. Pale, cool skin.
    C. Chest and back pain.
    D. Hematuria.
       1. A, C.
       2. B, C.
       3. A, D.
       4. B, D.

14. Match food from Column B to the appropriate diet in Column A.

Column A	Column B
____ 1. High sodium	A. Fish
____ 2. High potassium	B. Cereal
____ 3. High iron	C. Maple syrup
____ 4. High residue	D. Beef
____ 5. Low residue	E. Shellfish
____ 6. High protein	F. Organ meats
____ 7. High cholesterol	G. Banana
____ 8. Simple carbohydrate	H. Egg yolk

ANSWERS

1. CORRECT ANSWER IS 1
   Although identifying food preferences is helpful when planning a patient's menu, it is not an essential component of a nutritional assessment.
   (Page 397)

2. CORRECT ANSWER IS 3
   The patient should be encouraged to hold finger foods and fluid containers in order to assist with the feeding.
   (Page 401)

3. CORRECT ANSWER IS 2
   This diet will control the end products of protein metabolism and prevent ammonia buildup as well as decrease fluid accumulation.
   (Page 402)

4. CORRECT ANSWER IS 4
   This diet prevents accumulation of electrolytes and byproducts of metabolism.
   (Page 404)

5. CORRECT ANSWER IS 2
   Fat soluble vitamins are A, D, E, K. Whole milk, fortified margarine, and yellow and green leafy vegetables contain high levels of fat soluble vitamins.
   (Page 404)

6. CORRECT ANSWER IS 3
   Apples and fish are high in potassium while white-enriched and French bread, dry cereal, and pasta are foods low in potassium.
   (Page 405)

7. CORRECT ANSWER IS 2
   A daily intake of 2800 calories is required for usual/general tissue repair, whereas 6000 calories may be required for extensive tissue repair.
   (Page 406)

8. CORRECT ANSWER IS 4
   This measurement determines the appropriate length for tube insertion.
   (Page 409)

9. CORRECT ANSWER IS 3
   Listening over the stomach with a stethoscope while inserting 10 mL of air through the nasogastric tube is the best method when you do not have a choice of aspirating stomach contents and checking with litmus paper to determine if contents are acidic.
   (Page 409)

10. CORRECT ANSWER IS 1
    Use gentle pressure when irrigating a nasogastric tube to prevent damage to the stomach wall. Saline will prevent electrolyte imbalance.
    (Page 410)

11. CORRECT ANSWER IS 2
    The aspirate contains electrolytes and hydrochloric acid; therefore, it needs to be replaced to prevent an imbalance. With a residual of 50 mL, the usual action is to administer the tube feeding.
    (Page 410)

12. CORRECT ANSWER IS 3
    Checking for urine glucose is essential to prevent hyperosmolar situations.
    (Page 417)

13. CORRECT ANSWER IS 1
    Flushing, chest pain, and back pain are symptoms associated with lipid infusion side effects. Other symptoms include allergic responses.
    (Page 421)

14. CORRECT ANSWERS: 1=E, 2=G, 3=H, 4=B, 5=A, 6=D, 7=F, 8=C.
    (Pages 403–405)

Chapter Eighteen
Specimen Collection

QUESTIONS

1. The most important nursing action to maintain sterility of the urine container is to
   1. Wash the outside of the container with alcohol.
   2. Place container cap with sterile side down on 4 × 4 gauze.
   3. Avoid touching the inside of the container.
   4. Hold the container in an upright position.

2. You are asked to instruct a male patient in the procedure for obtaining a 24-hour urine specimen. Which one of the following instructions would be inappropriate to include?
   1. Cleanse the end of the penis with cleansing solution.
   2. Discard the first voided urine specimen.
   3. Collect the last voided specimen 24 hours after the first specimen.
   4. Discard the specimen collection if a small amount of urine is lost accidentally.

3. Collecting a stool specimen from an infant requires which of the following equipment?
   A. Cloth diaper.
   B. Plastic diaper liner.
   C. Cotton swabs.
   D. Sterile bedpan.
   E. Sterile glass container.
   1. A, B, D, E.
   2. B, C, E.
   3. A, B, C.
   4. All of the above.

4. The best time to collect a stool specimen for pinworms is
   1. Early morning.
   2. Late at night.
   3. After the bath.
   4. After lunch.

5. Jane has been ordered to have blood work drawn for serum electrolytes. She is on bed rest and has an IV in the basilic vein of the right forearm. The most appropriate site for blood withdrawal is
   1. Left upper arm (brachial vein).
   2. Right forearm (radial vein).
   3. Foot (greater saphenous vein).
   4. Left forearm (median cubital vein).

6. The tourniquet should be placed _____ before attempting to withdraw blood.
   1. Above the elbow
   2. Below the elbow
   3. Above the ankle
   4. Above the wrist

7. Place in sequence the steps for obtaining a blood specimen when measuring glucose via an autolet.
   A. Massage base of finger toward puncture site.
   B. Place recessed surface of platform against finger.
   C. Place a large drop of blood on both zones of Chemstrip.
   D. Match color chart for results.
   E. Wipe blood from the Chemstrip with dry cotton balls.
   1. A, B, C, E, D.
   2. A, B, C, D, E.
   3. B, A, E, C, D.
   4. B, A, C, E, D.

8. When obtaining a throat culture, the applicator stick is placed in a culture tube, allowed to sit for a few minutes in the medium to collect organisms, and discarded. Then, the culture tube is sent to the laboratory.
   1. True.
   2. False.

9. The most common reason for inaccurate reporting of a urine culture and sensitivity is

   1. Specimen sent to lab in unsterile container.
   2. Specimen not sent to lab immediately after collection.
   3. Cleansing agent not appropriate.
   4. Contaminated specimen.

10. When using the Accu-Chek, the screen displays HHH. This indicates

    1. The test is inaccurate and needs to be repeated.
    2. An insufficient blood droplet was placed on the test pad.
    3. The blood glucose is over 400 mg/dL.
    4. The battery is low and needs to be replaced.

ANSWERS

1. CORRECT ANSWER IS 3
Touching the inside of the container with your fingers or other objects will contaminate it. The cap is placed sterile side up on a firm surface.
(Page 431)

2. CORRECT ANSWER IS 1
The penis should be cleansed when obtaining a midstream specimen for a culture, not a 24-hour specimen.
(Page 431)

3. CORRECT ANSWER IS 3
A sterile bedpan is not required because the patient is an infant. A waxed cardboard box is used to send the specimen to the lab.
(Page 436)

4. CORRECT ANSWER IS 1
It is best to collect the stool specimen in the morning before the patient has defecated or bathed.
(Page 437)

5. CORRECT ANSWER IS 4
Blood should be drawn from the most peripheral vein to preserve the integrity of the vein for future lab work. With an IV in the right forearm, this site would be unacceptable for blood withdrawal.
(Page 438)

6. CORRECT ANSWER IS 1
Placing a tourniquet above the elbow will assist in vein distention for ease in specimen collection.
(Page 438)

7. CORRECT ANSWER IS 4
The finger is placed against the platform for the puncture. Massaging the base of the finger will assist in forming a large drop of blood, which is then placed on the Chemstrip.
(Page 440)

8. CORRECT ANSWER IS 2
The applicator stick is placed in the culture medium and sent to the laboratory.
(Page 446)

9. CORRECT ANSWER IS 4
Contaminated specimens can occur from improper cleansing or touching the top or inside of the container.
(Page 431)

10. CORRECT ANSWER IS 3
When the screen displays HHH, it indicates a blood glucose over 400 mg/dL. When the blood glucose registers at a high level, the test should be repeated.
(Page 442)

Chapter Nineteen
Diagnostic Tests

QUESTIONS

1. Patients undergoing contrast media studies should be observed closely for
   1. Constipation following studies.
   2. Hypertension.
   3. Hives and urticaria.
   4. Severe headache.

2. Following injections of iodine dye, the following diagnostic tests should not be performed because they show abnormal findings for 16 hours.
   A. Upper GI series.
   B. Urine sodium.
   C. 24-hour urine collection.
   D. Specific gravity.
   1. All except C.
   2. All except A.
   3. All except B.
   4. All of the above.

3. Nursing interventions for a patient scheduled for an oral cholecystogram would include
   1. Administering the iodine tablets the morning of the test.
   2. Ensuring that sufficient water is taken in the morning.
   3. Asking about allergies to food.
   4. Injecting the radiopaque dye the night before the study.

4. Nursing actions for a patient scheduled for an IVP include
   1. Giving a bland diet the night before.
   2. Restricting fluid intake after 6 PM the night before.
   3. Obtaining a consent form.
   4. Giving an enema just prior to the study.

5. Post cardiac catheterization care includes which of the following interventions?
   A. Check proximal pulses.
   B. Keep catheterization site extremity elevated.
   C. Restrict fluid intake for 24 hours.
   D. Apply pressure dressing to puncture site.
   1. A and C.
   2. B and D.
   3. B and C.
   4. All except A.

6. Instructions to the patient undergoing a lung scan should include
   1. Monitoring will take 2 hours after the IV injection of radioactive material.
   2. Radioactive gas is instilled by inhaling gas through an open system.
   3. Positions will be changed frequently to obtain clear images.
   4. The radioactive dye is administered orally the evening before the scan.

7. The purpose of completing a thallium scan with exercise is to
   1. Detect normal and healthy cells.
   2. Detect a recent MI.
   3. Identify myocardial scarring.
   4. Demonstrate perfusion problems not apparent when patient is at rest.

8. Barium studies are usually completed prior to arteriograms because barium interferes with the dye.
   1. True.
   2. False.

9. Patients are positioned on the left side following a liver biopsy.
   1. True
   2. False

10. Following a paracentesis, your patient's dressing is wet with serosanguineous fluid. Your initial intervention is to
    1. Place patient in shock position.
    2. Obtain vital signs.
    3. Notify physician.
    4. Change the dressing.

11. Instructions for a patient undergoing an arteriogram include
    1. "You may need to hold your breath when x-rays are taken."
    2. "You will be given a light anesthesia agent before the test."
    3. "Contrast media is not used for this procedure."
    4. "Ambulation is allowed upon return to the nursing unit."

12. The Queckenstedt's test is used to identify the
    1. Patency of arteries in the heart.
    2. Blockage of CSF flow in the subarachnoid space.
    3. Appropriate placement of the Trocar for a paracentesis.
    4. Iliac crest site for the bone marrow aspiration.

13. A priority nursing intervention following a gastroscopy is to
    1. Observe urine output every 2 hours.
    2. Medicate frequently for pain.
    3. Assess for gag reflex for 2 to 3 hours.
    4. Force fluids to eliminate the contrast media.

ANSWERS

1. CORRECT ANSWER IS 3
   Allergy to the iodine-based contrast media commonly manifests with hives, urticaria, nausea, and vomiting.
   (Page 453)

2. CORRECT ANSWER IS 2
   The dye is excreted through the urine; therefore, any urine test would be abnormal.
   (Page 456)

3. CORRECT ANSWER IS 3
   Allergies to food, particularly shellfish, should be identified and the physician notified since the patient will probably exhibit an allergic response to the dye.
   (Page 456)

4. CORRECT ANSWER IS 3
   A signed consent form is usually obtained for contrast media studies.
   (Page 456)

5. CORRECT ANSWER IS 2
   Keeping the affected extremity elevated prevents thrombus formation. Pressure dressings prevent bleeding.
   (Page 458)

6. CORRECT ANSWER IS 3
   Several position changes will allow for clear images of the lung fields.
   (Page 461)

7. CORRECT ANSWER IS 4
   Answers 1 and 3 refer to a thallium scan without exercise; answer 2 refers to a technetium pyrophosphate scan.
   (Page 462)

8. CORRECT ANSWER IS 2
   Barium studies are done following arteriograms because barium interferes with visualization of other structures.
   (Page 464)

9. CORRECT ANSWER IS 2
Patients are positioned on the right side to provide pressure and thus hemostasis of the liver.
(Page 468)

10. CORRECT ANSWER IS 4
This is to be expected as fluid will seep through the puncture site.
(Page 469)

11. CORRECT ANSWER IS 1
Patients may be instructed to hold their breath while x-rays are taken. Contrast media is used to allow for good visualization of the vessel. Bedrest is maintained for about 12 hours following the test. Premedication may be ordered, but patients are not given an anesthetic.
(Page 457)

12. CORRECT ANSWER IS 2
The Queckenstedt's test is used to identify blockage of CSF flow in the spinal subarachnoid space. When neck pressure is applied, a rapid rise in pressure level on the manometer occurs, with a return to normal within seconds.
(Page 467)

13. CORRECT ANSWER IS 3
Local anesthesia is used prior to the endoscope being inserted. The gag reflex returns in 2 to 3 hours. Until the reflex returns, foods and fluids must be withheld.
(Page 471)

Chapter Twenty
Urine Elimination

QUESTIONS

1. All of the following actions could be used to stimulate voiding except
   1. Putting oil of wintergreen on a cotton ball in the bedpan.
   2. Placing a hot washcloth on the patient's abdomen.
   3. Ambulating the patient.
   4. Placing the patient in a sitz bath.

2. Intake and output records include all of the following data except
   1. Blood transfusions.
   2. Nasogastric drainage.
   3. IV fluids.
   4. Enteral fluids.

3. Which one of the following statements about urine specific gravity is correct?
   1. The normal range is 1.020–1.030.
   2. The reading is taken at the fluid level on the side of the cylinder.
   3. The reading is taken when the urinometer is not moving for a more accurate result.
   4. The urinometer is spun so that it does not touch the side of the cylinder before the reading is taken.

4. The difference between the two-drop and the five-drop method for determining urine glucose is that the
   1. Five-drop method can be used only with adult patients.
   2. Five-drop method measures urine glucose to a 5% level.
   3. Two-drop method allows for a more definitive range in glucose levels.
   4. Second voided urine specimen is required only for the two-drop method.

5. You have been assigned to Mrs. Franks, who needs to have a sterile urine specimen sent to the laboratory for a culture and sensitivity. Which of the following items of equipment are necessary for catheterizing?
   A. Size 20 Foley catheter.
   B. Closed drainage bag and tubing.
   C. Clean gloves.
   D. Size 14 French catheter.
   E. Betadine solution.
   F. K-Y jelly.
   1. D, E, F.
   2. B, C, D.
   3. A, B, E, F.
   4. B, D, E, F.

6. You proceed to catheterize Mrs. Franks. After placing the sterile absorbent pad under the patient, what is the next action?
   1. Place outer white wrap under the patient's buttocks.
   2. Put on sterile gloves.
   3. Open sterile catheter package.
   4. Pour antiseptic solution over cotton balls.

7. After inserting the catheter, you find that urine is not flowing. Your next action is to
   1. Remove the catheter, check the meatus, and reinsert the catheter.
   2. Obtain a new, larger sized catheter and insert it.
   3. Reassess if catheter is in the vagina; if so, remove and reinsert into meatus.
   4. Insert the catheter a little farther, wait a few seconds, and if urine does not flow, reassess placement.

53

Review Questions Chapter Twenty

8. When the urine begins to flow through Mrs. Frank's catheter, your next action is to
   1. Inflate the catheter balloon with sterile water.
   2. Place the catheter tip into the specimen container.
   3. Connect the catheter into the drainage tubing.
   4. Place the catheter tip into the urine collection receptacle.

9. When providing catheter care for a patient with a retention catheter, the catheter is pulled taut and then cleansed with an antiseptic soaked cotton ball. Cleansing is started at the catheter insertion site and proceeds 5 inches down the catheter.
   1. True.
   2. False.

10. For patients with a suprapubic catheter, instructions for clamping protocol should include asking the patient to void when his bladder feels full.
   1. True.
   2. False.

11. The total amount of solution used to irrigate a catheter by opening a closed system or by irrigating a closed system is the same.
   1. True.
   2. False.

12. The flow rate of the irrigating solution used for continuous bladder irrigation is set at 40 to 60 drops per minute until it is discontinued.
   1. True.
   2. False.

13. Two important goals for Foley catheter care are maintaining sterility and providing for continuous urinary drainage. Which of the following nursing measures would NOT contribute to goal achievement?
   1. Keeping the urinary drainage bag below the level of the bed.
   2. Clamping off the catheter with a sterile plug when the patient is ambulating.
   3. Taking a urine culture and sensitivity by inserting a needle and syringe directly into the catheter.
   4. Irrigating the Foley only if complications occur.

14. If you have a physician's order to irrigate the bladder, which one of the following nursing measures will ensure patency?
   1. Use a solution of sterile water for the irrigation.
   2. Apply a small amount of pressure to push the mucus out of the catheter tip if the tube is not patent.
   3. Carefully insert about 100 mL of aqueous Zephiran into the bladder, allow it to remain for one hour, and then siphon it out.
   4. Irrigate with 30 mLs of normal saline to establish patency.

15. Mrs. Green's surgeon orders a Foley catheter to be inserted. Which one of the following interventions would you carry out first?
   1. Clean the perineum from front to back.
   2. Check the catheter for patency.
   3. Explain to Mrs. Green that she will feel slight, temporary discomfort.
   4. Arrange the sterile items on the sterile field.

ANSWERS

1. CORRECT ANSWER IS 3
Ambulating a patient stimulates flatus but does not stimulate voiding.
(Page 481)

2. CORRECT ANSWER IS 1
Blood is not considered a fluid replacement; therefore, it is not counted as fluid intake. Blood is recorded on a special section of the graphic sheet or on a special form.
(Page 481)

3. CORRECT ANSWER IS 4
The reading is taken just before the urinometer stops spinning and not if it is against the side of the cylinder.
(Page 483)

4. CORRECT ANSWER IS 3
The two-drop method chart shows seven colors in a scale ranging from 0–5%. The five-drop method has a range of four levels, 1+ to 4+, or 2%.
(Page 485)

5. CORRECT ANSWER IS 1
A urine specimen for culture and sensitivity requires catheterizing with a French (straight) catheter, cleansing the meatus with Betadine solution, and lubricating with K-Y jelly prior to insertion.
(Page 488)

6. CORRECT ANSWER IS 2
Sterile gloves are required to pour antiseptic solution over cotton balls. The catheter is contained in the package and does not have to be opened separately.
(Page 488)

7. CORRECT ANSWER IS 4
Check if catheter is inserted far enough into urethra or if it is in the vagina. If in vagina, leave in place as a landmark, obtain new sterile set-up, and insert new catheter.
(Page 494)

8. CORRECT ANSWER IS 2
When urine begins to flow, the catheter tip is placed into the specimen container. When the specimen is collected, the catheter tip is placed into the collection receptacle until urine flow ceases.
(Page 492)

9. CORRECT ANSWER IS 1
This procedure is correct as stated.
(Page 493)

10. CORRECT ANSWER IS 1
This promotes a normal voiding pattern in preparation for catheter removal.
(Page 498)

11. CORRECT ANSWER IS 1
The open and closed systems use the same amount of solution. The major difference is the opening of the closed system for irrigation, which leads to possible contamination.
(Page 501)

12. CORRECT ANSWER IS 2
The irrigation flow rate with clear drainage is 40–60 drops; otherwise, the rate is adjusted to the color and consistency of the urine. When the urine contains clots and is bright red, the flow rate is increased.
(Page 503)

13. CORRECT ANSWER IS 2
It is not acceptable to clamp the catheter when ambulating. The patient is instructed to keep the urinary bag below the bladder level. There is no need to open the system to obtain a sterile specimen.
(Page 496)

14. CORRECT ANSWER IS 4
It is never advisable to force fluids into tubing to check for patency. Sterile water and aqueous Zephiran will affect the pH of the bladder as well as cause irritation.
(Page 501)

15. CORRECT ANSWER IS 3
Giving the patient an adequate explanation for the procedure will result in less anxiety and more cooperation.
(Page 488)

Chapter Twenty-One
Bowel Elimination

QUESTIONS

1. Jason Barb, a 60-year-old patient, had abdominal surgery 2 days ago. He is complaining of severe "gas pains." The physician ordered the insertion of a rectal tube. The most appropriate rectal tube for Mr. Barb is a _____.

   1. 12 French
   2. 12 Foley
   3. 22 French
   4. 22 Foley

2. Mr. Barb is placed on his _____ side in a _____ position.

   1. Left side, recumbent
   2. Left side, Sims'
   3. Right side, semi-Fowler's
   4. Left side, semi-Fowler's

3. The tube is left in place _____ minutes.

   1. 10
   2. 20
   3. 30
   4. 60

4. A tap-water enema is ordered for Mr. Barb. The amount of fluid you will most likely administer is

   1. 250–300 mL.
   2. 300–500 mL.
   3. 500–750 mL.
   4. 750–1000 mL.

5. The temperature of the enema solution should be _____ °F.

   1. 95–100
   2. 100–105
   3. 105–110
   4. 110–120

6. The height of the water container should be _____ inches above the rectum.

   1. 10
   2. 18
   3. 20
   4. 24

7. The type of patients more at risk for complications when fecal impactions are removed include those with a

   1. CVA.
   2. Diagnosis requiring long-term bed rest.
   3. Permanent pacemaker.
   4. Spinal cord injury.

8. After removing the fecal impaction, the patient complains of feeling light-headed and the pulse rate is 44. Your priority intervention is to

   1. Monitor vital signs.
   2. Place in shock position.
   3. Call the physician.
   4. Begin CPR.

9. The rectal suppository is inserted beyond the rectal anal ridge.

   1. True.
   2. False.

10. You are developing a plan of care for a patient 3 days post-op with a permanent colostomy. He is ambulating and beginning to provide his own care. Your assessment should include which of the following essential factors?

A. The degree of mental alertness.
B. Whether he is right- or left-handed.
C. His bowel habits prior to surgery.
D. The amount of abdominal distention.
 1. A, C.
 2. C, D.
 3. All but B.
 4. All but C.

11. Which one of the following statements is most correct regarding colostomy irrigations?

1. The solution temperature should be 100°F.
2. 1000 mL is the usual amount of solution for the irrigation.
3. The solution container should be placed 10 inches above the stoma.
4. The irrigation cone is inserted in an upward direction in relation to the stoma.

12. Charting for colostomy irrigations should include

A. Condition of skin.
B. Amount of solution returned.
C. Color of stoma.
D. Circumference of pouch opening.
 1. A, B.
 2. B, C.
 3. All except D.
 4. All of the above.

ANSWERS

1. CORRECT ANSWER IS 3
The larger sized French catheter provides the best relief for flatus in adult patients.
(Page 533)

2. CORRECT ANSWER IS 1
The left side position assists in easy insertion of the tube due to the anatomical position of the rectum.
(Page 533)

3. CORRECT ANSWER IS 2
Prolonged stimulation of the anal sphincter may result in loss of neuromuscular response.
(Page 533)

4. CORRECT ANSWER IS 4
750 mL to 1000 mL is necessary to provide adequate stimulation for bowel evacuation.
(Page 539)

5. CORRECT ANSWER IS 3
This temperature prevents damage to tissues and abdominal cramping.
(Page 538)

6. CORRECT ANSWER IS 2
This height prevents too rapid instillation of the fluid, which may lead to cramping.
(Page 539)

7. CORRECT ANSWER IS 4
Spinal cord injured patients can affect a vagal response from manual removal of feces resulting in bradycardia.
(Page 535)

8. CORRECT ANSWER IS 2
The patient requires treatment for shock. Vital signs are monitored after placing the patient in the shock position; then the physician is called for orders.
(Page 535)

9. CORRECT ANSWER IS 1
The suppository will not be expelled as easily when it is inserted beyond the ridge.
(Page 536)

10. CORRECT ANSWER IS 3
Whether the patient is right- or left-handed is not important knowledge for providing care. The other factors are essential for beginning to plan a teaching program for the patient.
(Page 544)

11. CORRECT ANSWER IS 2
The same amount of irrigating solution is used for both an enema and a colostomy irrigation. The principle for both interventions is basically the same.
(Page 544)

12. CORRECT ANSWER IS 3
The circumference of the pouch opening is not essential information to chart. The pouch is cut 1/6 to 1/8 inch larger than the stoma.
(Page 546)

Chapter Twenty-Two
Heat and Cold Therapy

QUESTIONS

1. During your assessment, which of the following symptoms would indicate complications from heat treatments?

   A. Flushed face.
   B. Hypotension.
   C. Palpitations.
   D. Confusion.
   1. A, C.
   2. A, B, C.
   3. A, C, D.
   4. B, D.

2. When applying hot moist packs, your next action, after lubricating the skin with petroleum jelly, is to

   1. Check the skin for redness.
   2. Place the moist pack over unaffected area to check for heat tolerance.
   3. Place a moisture-proof pad under affected area.
   4. Place towels over affected area.

3. The steps in preparing for clean moist compresses include gathering the material, taking baseline vital signs, and lubricating the skin. The next step is to

   1. Inspect the skin for possible complications from the heat treatments.
   2. Place the compress material in a warming solution.
   3. Wring out the compresses.
   4. Put on sterile gloves.

4. The sitz bath procedure takes 20 minutes and during that time the patient should be assessed for vertigo, faintness, and weakness.

   1. True.
   2. False.

5. A heat lamp should be placed _____ inches from the patient and you should use no more than a _____ watt bulb.

   1. 18, 50
   2. 12, 25
   3. 18, 100
   4. 24, 60

6. An infant warmer is used in the newborn nursery to ensure maintenance of adequate body temperature. The major safety factor involved with the use of the warmer is to

   1. Ensure warmer is on manual control.
   2. Tape thermometer skin probe in place.
   3. Inspect skin under temperature probe at routine intervals.
   4. Adjust temperature of warmer each day to ensure it is set at 102°F.

7. For proper function of the aquathermic pad, which one of the following actions must be carried out?

   1. The reservoir container must be full at all times.
   2. The reservoir container must be kept below the bed for adequate water circulation.
   3. The pad is covered with a bath blanket to maintain heat to a specified body area.
   4. The pad is placed on an extremity with Kerlix gauze or tape to secure in place.

8. When administering a tepid bath, a patient begins to shiver. Your intervention should be to

   1. Continue with the bath, as this helps dissipate the heat.
   2. Stop the bath for a few minutes and place a warm blanket on the patient to stop shivering.
   3. Stop the bath, as the body is attempting to produce heat.
   4. Warm the solution, continue the bath, and change the location of cloth placement.

9. During an assessment, you find the patient's skin is irritated from the continuous use of an ice glove application. Your nursing action is to

   1. Massage the skin to bring blood to the area.
   2. Massage the whole area to warm it.
   3. Place a towel between the body area and the ice glove.
   4. Place the ice glove on an alternate body surface.

10. The hypothermia blanket is placed on a patient whose body temperature is 105°F. The most accurate statement about the blanket use is

    1. The blanket temperature should be started at 37°C and lowered every 15 minutes.
    2. Vital signs are monitored every 2 hours while reducing the temperature.
    3. Patients are placed on bath blankets that cover the cooling pad.
    4. The temperature probe is placed on the outer skin surface of the chest or abdomen.

ANSWERS

1. CORRECT ANSWER IS 1
   These are symptoms caused by vasodilation of blood vessels. Diaphoresis can also be observed as a complication of a heat treatment.
   (Page 563)

2. CORRECT ANSWER IS 3
   This action keeps the bed dry when the moist packs are applied. The moist towels are placed directly on the affected area and tested for response to heat.
   (Page 563)

3. CORRECT ANSWER IS 3
   The next step is to wring out the compress. Inspecting the skin and placing compresses in the warming solution are done prior to taking vital signs. Sterile gloves are not necessary.
   (Page 565)

4. CORRECT ANSWER IS 1
   These assessment modalities can occur as a result of vasodilation from the temperature (105 degrees to 110 degrees) of the water.
   (Page 566)

5. CORRECT ANSWER IS 4
   These safety measures prevent burning of the skin.
   (Page 568)

6. CORRECT ANSWER IS 3
   The probe can cause irritation. If this occurs, the probe is placed in a different location. An infant's skin is very delicate and becomes irritated easily.
   (Page 569)

7. CORRECT ANSWER IS 4
   Tape, not safety pins, is used to secure pads, as pins may puncture the material. Reservoirs are two-thirds filled and placed at bed level for adequate water circulation.
   (Page 570)

8. CORRECT ANSWER IS 3
   Stop or modify the bath to prevent shivering. Shivering is a method of producing body heat.
   (Page 573)

9. CORRECT ANSWER IS 4
After applying petroleum jelly to a different body area, apply the ice glove and observe for skin irritation. Massaging causes tissue damage.
(Page 574)

10. CORRECT ANSWER IS 1
The temperature of the cooling blanket is lowered every 15 minutes until 33 or 34°C temperature is reached.
(Page 576)

Chapter Twenty-Three
Wound Care

QUESTIONS

1. A nursing diagnosis pertinent to the care of a patient requiring wound care is

    1. Health Maintenance, Altered.
    2. Tissue Perfusion, Altered.
    3. Grieving, dysfunctional.
    4. Self-care deficit.

2. When picking up the first sterile glove from the package, pick it up by placing your nondominant hand under the folded cuff.

    1. True.
    2. False.

3. Sterile gloves can be adjusted to the hands for a better fit by maintaining the principle of "sterile surface to sterile surface."

    1. True.
    2. False.

4. When pouring a liquid from a sterile container, you should complete all of the following actions EXCEPT

    1. Place the bottle cap in an inverted fashion on the sterile field to prevent contamination.
    2. Pour a small amount of liquid into a nonsterile container before pouring it into the sterile container.
    3. Keep the label on the bottle facing upward when pouring into the container.
    4. Do not allow the bottle to touch the container when pouring liquids.
    5. Choose the statement that reflects an incorrect guideline for setting up a sterile field.
        1. Never turn your back on a sterile field.
        2. Keep sterile objects above waist level.
        3. You may reach across, but not touch a sterile field.
        4. Do not spill solutions on the sterile field.

6. When cleansing the skin surrounding an infected wound, start at the periphery and cleanse toward the wound.

    1. True.
    2. False.

7. To protect the skin under a drainage site, apply petroleum jelly and sterile gauze dressings under the drain.

    1. True.
    2. False.

8. Safety pins placed in drains should be cleaned frequently, for they cannot be replaced if they become encrusted.

    1. True.
    2. False.

9. Abdominal binders are wrapped at the time of surgery and rewrapped with dressing changes.

    1. True.
    2. False.

10. Wound drainage is only estimated when a hemovac suction is placed in a wound, as the system must remain closed.

    1. True.
    2. False.

11. Your patient suddenly coughs and an evisceration of the wound occurs. Your priority intervention is to

    1. Apply butterfly tape to the wound edges.
    2. Apply abdominal binder to the incision.
    3. Obtain vital signs.
    4. Place the patient in a supine position.

12. Wet-to-damp dressings require the use of a sterile solution soaked gauze dressing and clean surgical gloves.

1. True.
2. False.

13. Pressure ulcers occur in stages according to the degree of skin involvement. Specific treatments are advised for each stage.

1. True.
2. False.

ANSWERS

1. CORRECT ANSWER IS 2
Blood supply may be altered to the wound area leading to an alteration in tissue perfusion.
(Page 585)

2. CORRECT ANSWER IS 2
The glove is picked up by the folded edge of cuff, using the nondominant hand.
(Page 587)

3. CORRECT ANSWER IS 1
Keeping sterile surfaces of the gloves in contact with each other will allow gloves to be adjusted without contamination occurring.
(Page 587)

4. CORRECT ANSWER IS 1
The bottle cap is placed in an inverted position on a clean, firm surface to prevent contamination. It is not placed on the sterile field.
(Page 588)

5. CORRECT ANSWER IS 3
You should avoid reaching across a sterile field as well as touching it, so that it does not become contaminated.
(Page 590)

6. CORRECT ANSWER IS 1
For dirty wounds, the cleansing procedure starts at the periphery and moves toward the wound. With clean wounds, the cleansing starts at the incision site and moves toward the periphery.
(Page 593)

7. CORRECT ANSWER IS 1
Petroleum jelly and sterile dressings provide protection for the skin under drains.
(Page 595)

8. CORRECT ANSWER IS 2
When safety pins become encrusted, they should be replaced with sterile safety pins.
(Page 594)

9. CORRECT ANSWER IS 2
Abdominal binders are rewrapped every 8 hours, but assessed every 4 hours for effectiveness.
(Page 595)

10. CORRECT ANSWER IS 2
Hemovac suctions are emptied every shift, and the drainage measured and documented.
(Page 597)

11. CORRECT ANSWER IS 4
The patient's wound opens and the bowel contents protrude when an evisceration occurs. Intra-abdominal pressure changes create a shock state; thus the supine position is required.
(Page 600)

12. CORRECT ANSWER IS 2
Sterile gloves are required for the dressing change, as this is considered a sterile procedure.
(Page 602)

13. CORRECT ANSWER IS 1
An increase in the amount of skin involvement requires specific interventions to promote healing.
(Page 602)

Chapter Twenty-Four
Respiratory Care

QUESTIONS

1. While instructing a patient in deep breathing exercises, you explain that he needs to
   1. Breathe in slowly through his mouth.
   2. Exhale slowly through pursed lips.
   3. Exhale rapidly through pursed lips.
   4. Breathe in slowly through his nose.

2. Instructions in the use of flow spirometers include
   1. Take a deep breath and then place mouth around the mouthpiece and exhale into spirometer.
   2. Hold spirometer at a right angle and breathe into mouthpiece.
   3. Keep the ball of the spirometer elevated for 3 seconds.
   4. Exhale into the mouthpiece to keep the ball elevated for 10 seconds.

3. Charting for deep breathing and coughing procedures would NOT be likely to include which of the following?
   1. Changes in pulse and respirations.
   2. Position in which procedures are done.
   3. Amount of secretions expectorated.
   4. Patient's participation in procedure.

4. Jamie, previously hospitalized for left lower lobe pneumonia, is now admitted for abdominal pain. Due to her respiratory history, the physician has requested several preventative interventions be carried out. Chest physiotherapy is ordered. Prior to providing this intervention, your priority action is to
   1. Instruct her in diaphragmatic breathing.
   2. Assess vital signs.
   3. Auscultate lung fields.
   4. Assess characteristics of her sputum.

5. Percussion is performed _____.
   1. Over each lung lobe for 1 minute
   2. On exhalation only
   3. By cupping the hands and clapping rhythmically
   4. By using the fingertips to put pressure on the lung segment

6. When performing naso-oral suctioning, the correct action is to
   1. Insert the catheter 6 to 8 inches into nares.
   2. Apply suction while inserting the catheter into the bronchus.
   3. Apply continuous suction as the catheter is removed during the procedure.
   4. Suction for 30 seconds and then allow a 3-minute rest period.

7. Signs of hypoxia occur during a suctioning procedure. The change in the procedure that can prevent hypoxia is to
   1. Ensure that the catheter is no more than three quarters the diameter of the tube.
   2. Limit suction time to 30 seconds.
   3. Hyperinflate lungs with 100% oxygen prior to suctioning.
   4. Suction no more than three consecutive times before administering oxygen.

8. When assessing if a patient needs oxygen therapy, you would be alert for which of the following clinical manifestations?
   A. Yawning.
   B. Bradycardia.
   C. Restlessness.
   D. Rosy lips.
   1. A, C.
   2. B, D.
   3. A, C, D.
   4. All of the above.

9. Your patient requires the highest possible concentration of oxygen. Which delivery system will you use?

   1. Nasal cannula.
   2. Venturi mask.
   3. Face tent.
   4. Mask with reservoir bag.

10. The procedure for maintaining oxygen delivery through a nasal cannula includes

    A. Start oxygen flow at 3 liters/minute.
    B. Insert catheter 8 inches into the nares.
    C. Observe patient for gastric distention.
    D. Attach oxygen tubing to a humidification system.
       1. A, B.
       2. B, C.
       3. A, C, D.
       4. B, D.

11. Nursing care and assessments for infants under an oxygen hood can be provided by opening the lid.

    1. True.
    2. False.

12. The most important nursing intervention for patients on IPPB therapy is to

    1. Make the patient comfortable in a supine position during the treatment.
    2. Monitor blood pressure, pulse, and respirations before and after the treatment.
    3. Instruct the patient to inhale, and then cover mouthpiece with mouth and exhale into the machine.
    4. Instruct the patient to breathe at the rate of 20 times per minute.

13. Equipment necessary for cleaning an inner cannula in a patient with a new tracheostomy includes

    A. Clean gloves.
    B. Second inner cannula.
    C. Hydrogen peroxide.
    D. Pipe cleaners.
       1. A, C.
       2. B, D.
       3. B, C, D.
       4. All of the above.

14. When changing trach ties without assistance, old ties are left in place until new ties are anchored.

    1. True.
    2. False.

15. A manual resuscitator bag is compressed every 5 seconds for an apneic adult patient.

    1. True.
    2. False.

16. Most tracheostomy cuffs are inflated with 15 mLs of air.

    1. True.
    2. False.

17. Thomas Mann was injured in an automobile accident. His thorax hit the steering wheel, which resulted in a tension pneumothorax. Thomas has chest tubes inserted. Which of the following nursing interventions should NOT be included in his care plan?

    1. Place hemostats on the bed as a safety measure in case of air leaks.
    2. Milk (or strip) the chest tubes every 2 to 4 hours to maintain patency.
    3. Report chest drainage in excess of 200 mL/hour to the physician.
    4. Keep Thomas flat in bed to avoid the formation of leaks and to promote drainage.

18. Nursing responsibilities associated with Thomas's chest tubes will include

    1. Keeping the chest tubes free of kinking and obstruction by coiling them loosely to the bed.
    2. Keeping the bottle at bed level to prevent backflow.
    3. Checking that water fluctuation is continuous in the trap bottle.
    4. Checking that the amount of pressure does not exceed 5 cm water in the pressure chamber.

19. While completing an assessment, you notice that fluid is fluctuating up and down in the long tube of the water-seal bottle. What is your initial intervention?

    1. Clamp the chest tubes closest to the patient.
    2. Call the physician immediately.
    3. Look for leaks in the tubing.
    4. Do nothing because this fluctuation is normal.

20. Continuous air bubbling in the water-seal bottle indicates that
    1. Air is passing out of the pleural space.
    2. Air is being removed from within the lung tissue.
    3. Air is leaking into the drainage system.
    4. Nothing is wrong, as air bubbling is normal.

21. Three-bottle suction and disposable water-seal systems use the same principles in function.
    1. True.
    2. False.

ANSWERS

1. CORRECT ANSWER IS 4
Breathing slowly through the nose and exhaling normally is the method of instruction for deep breathing exercises.
(Page 616)

2. CORRECT ANSWER IS 3
This action provides for alveolar inflation, which promotes gas exchange and mobilization of secretions.
(Page 617)

3. CORRECT ANSWER IS 2
Unless the position used for deep breathing and coughing is unusual, it is generally not charted.
(Page 618)

4. CORRECT ANSWER IS 3
Auscultating lung fields provides knowledge of which lung areas are most affected. These areas should be treated first, as many patients cannot tolerate a 30-minute procedure.
(Page 619)

5. CORRECT ANSWER IS 3
Cupping the hands and clapping over each lobe segment promotes mobilization of secretions.
(Page 620)

6. CORRECT ANSWER IS 1
The catheter is inserted through the nares without applying suction. Suctioning is limited to 15 seconds, and suction on the catheter is released intermittently during the procedure.
(Page 624)

7. CORRECT ANSWER IS 3
Hyperinflation of lungs with oxygen prevents hypoxia during suctioning procedure in patients requiring frequent treatments.
(Page 624)

8. CORRECT ANSWER IS 1
Hypoxia results in yawning, restlessness, shortness of breath, and tachycardia.
(Page 629)

9. CORRECT ANSWER IS 4
A mask with a reservoir bag provides 70–100% oxygen at flow rates of 8–10 liters.
(Page 630)

10. CORRECT ANSWER IS 3
Oxygen is started at 3 liters and attached to a humidification system. When mouth breathing results from cannula insertion into the nares, observe the patient for gastric distention.
(Page 632)

11. CORRECT ANSWER IS 1
This procedure avoids decreasing the oxygen level while nursing care is delivered.
(Page 635)

12. CORRECT ANSWER IS 2
Alterations in vital signs could be an indication of nebulizer medication side effects.
(Page 644)

13. CORRECT ANSWER IS 3
Sterile gloves are required for cleaning the inner cannula, especially for patients with a new tracheostomy.
(Page 646)

14. CORRECT ANSWER IS 1
It is a safe practice to keep the trach tube anchored with the old ties when changing them without assistance. This prevents the tube from being dislodged during the process.
(Page 648)

15. CORRECT ANSWER IS 1
This provides a respiratory rate of 12 per minute, which is necessary for tissue oxygenation.
(Page 651)

16. CORRECT ANSWER IS 2
Tracheostomy cuffs are generally inflated with 5 mLs of air.
(Page 684)

17. CORRECT ANSWER IS 4
Thomas should be placed in a semi-Fowler's or high-Fowler's position to assist with drainage and adequate ventilation.
(Page 657)

18. CORRECT ANSWER IS 1
This placement of the chest tubes prevents kinking.
(Page 656)

19. CORRECT ANSWER IS 4
This condition is expected. Water moves up the tube on inspiration and down the tube on expiration.
(Page 659)

20. CORRECT ANSWER IS 3
Bubbling in the water-seal bottle indicates an air leak somewhere in the system.
(Page 659)

21. CORRECT ANSWER IS 1
The systems function on the same principles of re-establishing negative pressure. The chambers in the disposable system are similar to the bottles.
(Page 660)

Chapter Twenty-Five
Circulatory Maintenance

QUESTIONS

1. Janet Moen comes to the emergency room with severe lacerations. While assessing her, you find that she is bleeding profusely from a deep laceration on her left lower forearm. Your first choice of action is to

   1. Apply a tourniquet just below the elbow.
   2. Apply pressure directly over the wound.
   3. Call for the physician to check the wound.
   4. Place Janet in shock position.

2. You are concerned when Janet continues to bleed even with direct pressure. Your next action is to

   1. Apply ice to lower the body temperature.
   2. Monitor closely for signs of shock.
   3. Elevate her upper extremities and apply blankets to raise her body temperature.
   4. Maintain a patent airway and prevent vomiting.

3. When measuring Mr. Hendel for knee-high elastic hose, you would measure his

   1. Leg length from heel to buttocks and calf circumference while he is standing.
   2. Ankle and calf circumference while he is standing.
   3. Leg length to the knee when he is lying down.
   4. Calf circumference and leg length from bottom of heel to bend of knee.

4. You have orders to apply rotating tourniquets to a patient in severe pulmonary edema. Nursing interventions carried out during the procedure would include all of the following EXCEPT

   1. Place patient in low-Fowler's position.
   2. Obtain baseline vital signs.
   3. Apply cuffs to the most proximal area of the extremity (toward the trunk).
   4. Mark pulse site for a reference point.

5. When rotating the tourniquet pressure, one cuff is inflated before the pressure is released in the next cuff.

   1. True.
   2. False.

6. Select the statement that correctly identifies a normal ECG strip.

   1. P-R interval falls before the QRS complex on the strip.
   2. T-wave should be in the inverted position on the strip.
   3. P-R interval should be no longer than .12 seconds.
   4. QRS interval should be no longer than .20 seconds.

7. A normal PR interval is no more than _____ seconds.

   1. 0.04
   2. 0.06
   3. 0.12
   4. 0.20

8. Normal QRS activity takes less than _____ seconds.

   1. 0.04
   2. 0.06
   3. 0.12
   4. 0.20

9. The PR interval represents the time it takes for the

   1. Impulse to begin atrial contraction.
   2. Impulse to traverse the atria to the AV node.
   3. SA node to discharge the impulse to begin atrial depolarization.
   4. Impulse to travel to the ventricles.

10. Place in sequence the steps for CPR protocol.

    A. Call "code."
    B. Check carotid pulse.
    C. Ventilate with two slow breaths.
    D. Begin resuscitation.
       1. B, C, D, A.
       2. D, C, B, A.
       3. A, C, B, D.
       4. B, A, D, C.

11. The ratio of CPR for an adult patient is

    1. 15:1 for one rescuer.
    2. 5:1 for two rescuers.
    3. 5:2 for two rescuers.
    4. 15:2 for two rescuers.

12. The compression rate for an infant requiring CPR is _____ per minute.

    1. 80
    2. 100
    3. 110
    4. 120

13. If aspiration of a foreign body is suspected and one attempt to ventilate is not successful, your next intervention is to

    1. Administer four quick breaths.
    2. Deliver four back blows.
    3. Deliver four abdominal thrusts.
    4. Reposition head and attempt to ventilate.

14. When performing a Heimlich maneuver, position your hands

    1. Over the xiphoid process.
    2. Just above the umbilicus.
    3. Halfway between xiphoid and umbilicus.
    4. Just under the xiphoid process.

ANSWERS

1. CORRECT ANSWER IS 2
   The first action is to apply direct pressure to the wound. If the bleeding continues, additional actions must be taken. They include placing her in shock position and perhaps applying a tourniquet.
   (Page 680)

2. CORRECT ANSWER IS 2
   Blood loss results in shock; therefore, close monitoring of vital signs and shock symptoms is essential.
   (Page 681)

3. CORRECT ANSWER IS 4
   Patient should be in dorsal recumbent position with bed elevated. For knee-high hose, measurement is taken from the Achilles' tendon to the popliteal fold and the mid-calf circumference.
   (Page 682)

4. CORRECT ANSWER IS 1
   To provide for lung expansion, the patient is placed in a high-Fowler's position.
   (Page 685)

5. CORRECT ANSWER IS 2
The cuff is always deflated first before the next cuff is inflated. A principle to remember is that all cuffs are never inflated at one time.
(Page 686)

6. CORRECT ANSWER IS 1
The P-R interval indicates atrial contraction; therefore, it should precede the QRS complex, which is indicative of ventricular contraction.
(Page 689)

7. CORRECT ANSWER IS 4
The normal range for the PR interval is 0.12 to 0.20 seconds.
(Page 689)

8. CORRECT ANSWER IS 3
The time required for ventricular conduction of the impulse is 0.04 to 0.12 seconds.
(Page 689)

9. CORRECT ANSWER IS 4
The PR interval is measured on the ECG strip from the beginning of the P wave to the beginning of the QRS complex.
(Page 689)

10. CORRECT ANSWER IS 3
A code is called after the "look, listen, and feel for breathing" action is taken; ventilation is then attempted.
(Page 694)

11. CORRECT ANSWER IS 2
When there are two rescuers, the procedure is to give one breath for each five chest compressions.
(Page 695)

12. CORRECT ANSWER IS 2
Cardiac compressions of 100 per minute should provide adequate circulation to vital organs.
(Page 695)

13. CORRECT ANSWER IS 4
Repositioning the head may be all that is required to open the airway.
(Page 697)

14. CORRECT ANSWER IS 3
This position assists in forcing the foreign body out of the trachea by making use of the residual air in the lungs.
(Page 697)

Chapter Twenty-Six
Intravenous Therapy

QUESTIONS

1. Essential equipment you need to gather for preparation of an IV system includes

    A. Metal IV tubing clamp.
    B. IV tubing with drip chamber.
    C. IV pole.
    D. Stopcock.
    1. B, C, D.
    2. B, C.
    3. A, B, C.
    4. All of the above.

2. Place in sequence the steps for preparing the IV solution using a plastic container.

    A. Close control clamp.
    B. Insert the spike into the port.
    C. Remove plastic protector from administration port.
    D. Remove outer wrap from IV bag.
    E. Invert IV container and release pressure on drip chamber.
    1. A, D, B, C, E.
    2. C, D, E, B, A.
    3. D, E, C, B, A.
    4. D, C, A, B, E.

3. In preparing an IV site, you hang the IV bag on the pole. The next step is to

    1. Cut the tape.
    2. Select a vein.
    3. Prepare site with povidone-iodine.
    4. Position the patient.

4. Dilating a vein in preparation for a venipuncture can be accomplished by all of the following interventions EXCEPT

    1. Have patient open and close fist several times.
    2. Instruct patient to elevate hand above heart.
    3. Apply warm compresses for 10 minutes.
    4. Apply tourniquet for 1 to 2 minutes.

5. Winged-tip needles are inserted into the vein at a 90-degree angle.

    1. True.
    2. False.

6. For easy insertion through the skin, the bevel of the needle is placed downward facing the skin.

    1. True.
    2. False.

7. When using an over-the-needle catheter, the needle is withdrawn from inside the catheter immediately after the needle enters the vein.

    1. True.
    2. False.

8. You have been assigned to care for Mrs. Clark, a 68-year-old patient with a CVA. She has an IV infusing at 50 mL per hour. The IV administration set delivers 15 gtts/mL. When adjusting the flow rate, you regulate the drops at _____ per minute.

    1. 4
    2. 8
    3. 12
    4. 25

9. The IV is placed on a controller to maintain the flow rate. If the alarm sounds on the controller, you will complete all of the following actions EXCEPT

    1. Ensure that the drip chamber is full.
    2. Assess that height of IV container is at least 30 inches above venipuncture site.
    3. Ensure that the drop sensor is properly placed on the drip chamber.
    4. Evaluate the needle and IV tubing to determine if they are patent and positioned appropriately.

10. While performing IV site care for Mrs. Clark, you assess the site for all of the following EXCEPT

1. Erythema.
2. Edema.
3. Serosanguineous fluid.
4. Infiltration.

11. When changing Mrs. Clark's gown, your first action is to untie it at the neck. The next step is to

1. Remove the IV bottle from the hook and slip the sleeve over the bottle.
2. Remove the gown from the unaffected arm.
3. Place a clean gown over the chest before attempting to remove the used gown.
4. Remove the gown from both arms at the same time.

12. Assessment of Mrs. Clark reveals a dehydrated state. Which of the following clinical manifestations are indicative of this state?

A. Taut, shiny skin.
B. Firm eyeballs.
C. Weak, thready pulse.
D. Dry, flaking skin.
  1. A, B, C.
  2. A, B.
  3. C, D.
  4. All of the above.

13. When administering IV medications, an additive bag/bottle is hung below the level of the primary bottle.

1. True.
2. False.

14. To maintain a patent heparin lock, a saline solution is injected into the needle and catheter between usage.

1. True.
2. False.

15. To determine that medication is inserted directly into the vein, inject the medication slowly and observe for unusual reactions surrounding the IV site.

1. True.
2. False.

16. To ensure that the correct blood transfusion is administered, the safety procedures include checking the

A. Blood unit number.
B. Patient's blood group and type.
C. Blood transfusion request form.
D. Patient's ID number.
  1. A, B.
  2. All except D.
  3. All except C.
  4. All of the above.

17. Blood is infused at _____ drops per minute for the first 15 minutes of the transfusion.

1. 10
2. 20
3. 30
4. 60

18. Janet needs to have an IV started in order to maintain the intravascular compartment and replace blood volume. Which of the following solutions will most likely be used to start the blood administration?

1. Lactated Ringer's solution.
2. D_5W.
3. Normal saline.
4. Albumin.

19. Janet was given several blood transfusions following surgery. Which one of the following clinical manifestations is an early indication of a transfusion reaction?

1. Urticaria.
2. Dyspnea.
3. Hematuria.
4. Cyanosis.

20. The normal CVP range is 10–20 cm water.

1. True.
2. False.

21. The purpose of using a heparin-filled tbc syringe for irrigating a nonpatent Hickman catheter is to increase pressure in the system.

1. True.
2. False.

22. Anyone who has frequent heparin flushes on an IV line should have prothrombin times checked frequently.

1. True.
2. False.

ANSWERS

1. CORRECT ANSWER IS 2
The IV administration set contains a plastic clamp on the set. A stopcock is not essential for the routine IV set-up.
(Page 706)

2. CORRECT ANSWER IS 4
The plastic outer wrap is removed from the container before the IV set-up can be prepared.
(Page 707)

3. CORRECT ANSWER IS 4
Position the patient in such a manner that he is comfortable and the IV site is easily observed.
(Page 711)

4. CORRECT ANSWER IS 2
To distend the veins, the arm needs to be placed in a dependent position, such as over the edge of the bed.
(Page 711)

5. CORRECT ANSWER IS 2
They are inserted at a 30- to 40-degree angle.
(Page 712)

6. CORRECT ANSWER IS 2
The bevel of the needle is placed upward to facilitate piercing the skin.
(Page 712)

7. CORRECT ANSWER IS 2
The needle is withdrawn after the catheter and needle are fully in place.
(Page 714)

8. CORRECT ANSWER IS 3
To calculate the drip factor, multiply the hourly rate times the drop factor (50 mL times 15). Divide the answer by 60 minutes (750/60 = 12.5 gtt/min). Round off answer to 12.
(Page 719)

9. CORRECT ANSWER IS 1
The drip chamber should be only one-third full so that the sensor can "pick up" the drops.
(Page 720)

10. CORRECT ANSWER IS 3
Serosanguineous fluid is expected from a drainage site or wound, not an IV site.
(Page 723)

11. CORRECT ANSWER IS 2
It is much easier to remove the gown by first taking it off the unaffected arm, as the IV bottle and tubing must be slipped through the gown on the affected side.
(Page 725)

12. CORRECT ANSWER IS 3
Responses C and D are present when a patient is dehydrated. Responses A and B are indicative of an overhydrated state.
(Page 729)

13. CORRECT ANSWER IS 2
The additive bag/bottle is hung above the level of the primary IV bottle to ensure that the primary bottle infuses fluid after the additive bag/bottle is empty.
(Page 733)

14. CORRECT ANSWER IS 2
A heparin lock is injected with a heparin solution to maintain a patent system between usage.
(Page 736)

15. CORRECT ANSWER IS 2
The plunger of the syringe is pulled back after the needle is inserted into the vein to observe for blood flashback. The medication is then injected into the vein.
(Page 737)

16. CORRECT ANSWER IS 4
All of the above safety checks are necessary to prevent administering a mismatched unit of blood.
(Page 741)

17. CORRECT ANSWER IS 2
This procedure allows adequate time to observe for possible blood reactions.
(Page 740)

18. CORRECT ANSWER IS 3
This solution prevents agglutination of RBCs because it contains electrolytes.
(Page 739)

19. CORRECT ANSWER IS 1
The earliest sign of a transfusion reaction involves the skin and includes urticaria, itching, and hives.
(Page 743)

20. CORRECT ANSWER IS 2
Normal CVP is 5–10 cm water.
(Page 750)

21. CORRECT ANSWER IS 1
A small syringe exerts more pressure on the system.
(Page 752)

22. CORRECT ANSWER IS 1
Heparin may cause serious side effects such as abnormal clotting or bleeding so frequent prothrombin times are necessary.
(Page 755)

Chapter Twenty-Seven
Orthopedic Measures

QUESTIONS

1. When treating a patient with a sprain or strain injury, you will
   1. Apply heat for 4 hours.
   2. Apply cold and heat alternating every hour for 24 hours.
   3. Apply cold for 4 hours.
   4. Apply cold for 24 to 48 hours.

2. The repair process following a bone fracture begins with
   1. The laying down of the organic matrix.
   2. Formation of a blood clot.
   3. Osteoblast formation.
   4. Fibroblast development.

3. A comminuted fracture is best defined as a
   1. Bone completely broken in a transverse, spiral, or oblique direction.
   2. Bone exposed to the air through a break in the skin.
   3. Fracture associated with soft tissue injuries.
   4. Bone broken with disruption of both sides of the periosteum.

4. Bryant's traction would most likely be used in which condition?
   1. Elderly patient with hip fracture prior to surgery.
   2. Cervical cord injury.
   3. Fractured femur in a toddler.
   4. Fractured tibia or fibula in young adolescents.

5. When applying a sling, place the apex, or point, of the triangle toward the _____ and bring the opposite end around the affected arm and _____.
   1. Wrist, anchor at neck
   2. Elbow, over affected shoulder
   3. Wrist, over affected shoulder
   4. Elbow, anchor at back of neck

6. When applying a circular bandage, begin the wrap by
   1. Anchoring the wrap at the distal end.
   2. Anchoring the wrap at the proximal end.
   3. Beginning the circular turn at the distal end.
   4. Beginning the circular turn at the proximal end.

7. An air splint can be deflated
   1. If frank bleeding is observed.
   2. Prior to x-rays.
   3. By nurses prior to assessing area.
   4. By physicians only.

8. The major differences between a plaster of Paris and a synthetic cast is that the
   1. Drying time is prolonged with a synthetic cast.
   2. Synthetic cast is less restrictive.
   3. Plaster cast requires expensive equipment for application.
   4. Synthetic cast is more effective for immobilizing severely displaced bones.

9. Assessment modalities for a patient with a casted extremity include
   A. Identifying an increase in drainage from a wound.
   B. Applying pressure to nailbed to observe color return.
   C. Asking the patient about coolness of cast.
   D. Checking on cleanliness of the cast.
   1. A and B.
   2. C and D.
   3. B and C.
   4. A and D.

10. Skeletal traction should be removed and skin care provided to the affected area every 4 hours.

   1. True.
   2. False.

11. While assessing a patient in skeletal traction, you observe the distal extremity to be pale with slow capillary refill and palpated a 1+ pulse. Your initial action is to

   1. Assess the patient every 15 minutes for changes.
   2. Observe for ecchymosis or signs of infection.
   3. Remove the traction.
   4. Notify physician.

12. Your assessment for a patient with an amputated limb should include range-of-motion and muscle strength capability.

   1. True.
   2. False.

ANSWERS

1. **CORRECT ANSWER IS 4**
   Ice decreases edema formation and thus helps minimize other complications.
   (Page 766)

2. **CORRECT ANSWER IS 2**
   Clot formation begins the repair process followed by osteoblasts and fibroblasts converging on the site and laying down the organic matrix.
   (Page 766)

3. **CORRECT ANSWER IS 1**
   A comminuted fracture can be broken into several fragments in addition to a transverse, spiral, or oblique direction.
   (Page 767)

4. **CORRECT ANSWER IS 3**
   Bryant's traction is a type of skin traction used for children under 3 years who have sustained a fractured femur.
   (Page 768)

5. **CORRECT ANSWER IS 2**
   After bringing the triangle toward the elbow, bring the sling around the affected arm and over the shoulder; then tie it at the side of the neck.
   (Page 771)

6. **CORRECT ANSWER IS 1**
   The bandage is anchored at the distal end using two circular turns and then beginning the wrap.
   (Page 772)

7. **CORRECT ANSWER IS 4**
   Once an air splint is applied, only a physician may deflate it.
   (Page 774)

8. **CORRECT ANSWER IS 2**
   A synthetic cast is less restrictive, lighter in weight, and requires less drying time than a plaster of Paris cast.
   (Page 776)

9. **CORRECT ANSWER IS 1**
   The assessment is based on circulation, motion, and sensation. Increased drainage can lead to skin excoriation. Slow capillary refill reflects decreased circulation to the area.
   (Page 777)

10. **CORRECT ANSWER IS 2**
    Skeletal traction is not removed. Only skin traction is removed.
    (Page 781)

11. CORRECT ANSWER IS 4
There is a circulatory compromise and thus the physician needs to be notified immediately. The other actions, except removing traction, will be carried out later.
(Page 781)

12. CORRECT ANSWER IS 1
Range-of-motion and muscle strength parameters can assist you to predict the patient's ability to get out of bed and crutch walk
(Page 785)

Chapter Twenty-Eight
Operative Care

QUESTIONS

1. The degree of anxiety and stress experienced at the time of surgery is dependent on the patient's

   A. Belief system.
   B. Number of prior surgeries.
   C. Type of surgical procedure.
   D. Degree of self-esteem.
   1. B and C.
   2. A and D.
   3. A, B, and D.
   4. All of the above.

2. Prolonged high-stress levels in the preoperative period can lead to which of the following conditions?

   A. Deficient immune system.
   B. Hypotension.
   C. Hyponatremia.
   D. Life-threatening arrhythmias.
   1. A and D.
   2. B and C.
   3. B, C, and D.
   4. All of the above.

3. When a patient becomes angry, your best intervention is to

   1. Isolate the patient until he calms down.
   2. Explore actions which will meet the patient's needs.
   3. Tell the patient to stop the behavior if he expects a response from you.
   4. Remove the patient from his room and take him to a quiet place.

4. Essential baseline data for surgical patients includes all of the following EXCEPT

   1. Physical assessment.
   2. Laboratory and ECG report.
   3. Patient teaching documentation.
   4. History of allergies.

5. Preoperative teaching by the nurse includes which of the following explanations?

   1. Discussion of surgical procedure.
   2. Complications of surgical procedure.
   3. Anesthetic drugs to be used.
   4. Discussion of equipment used postoperatively.

6. The surgical scrub should start at the periphery and move in a circular motion toward the incision site.

   1. True.
   2. False.

7. Patients at risk for postoperative infections include all of the following EXCEPT those who have a history of

   1. Previous surgeries.
   2. Obesity.
   3. Prolonged antibiotic therapy.
   4. Corticosteroid therapy.

8. The factor least likely to appear on the surgical check list is

   1. Vital signs.
   2. History.
   3. Allergies.
   4. Stress level of patient.

9. The surgical consent form includes all of the following information EXCEPT

   1. Name of procedure.
   2. Patient's signature.
   3. Date of procedure.
   4. Surgeon's signature.

10. Preoperative care charting should include
    A. Safety measures.
    B. Solution and length of time for surgical scrub.
    C. Information provided about surgery to patient.
    D. History of patient's need for surgery.
       1. A and B.
       2. All except A.
       3. All except D.
       4. All of the above.

11. The diet progression for patients with major surgery is
    1. Clear liquids upon return from surgery to soft diet first postoperative day.
    2. Soft diet after presence of bowel sounds.
    3. N.P.O. and then clear liquids when bowel sounds return.
    4. Clear liquids when awake, full liquids first postoperative day.

12. Atelectasis, a major postoperative complication, presents with which of the following findings?
    A. Tachypnea.
    B. Temperature of 99.6°F.
    C. Dullness to breath sound percussion.
    D. Restlessness.
       1. C only.
       2. A and D.
       3. All except B.
       4. All of the above.

ANSWERS

1. **CORRECT ANSWER IS 4**
   Although the impact depends on the patient's experience and how well the patient was prepared, the type of procedure and number of prior surgeries also influence the degree of anxiety and stress.
   (Page 803)

2. **CORRECT ANSWER IS 1**
   Arrhythmias result from electrolyte imbalances. A deficient immune system may result from prolonged stress. Water and sodium retention is a result of catecholamine release associated with stress.
   (Page 803)

3. **CORRECT ANSWER IS 2**
   This will help decrease his anger state, as most likely his needs are not being met. Do not reward his behavior or isolate him as this action is not therapeutic.
   (Page 808)

4. **CORRECT ANSWER IS 3**
   While patient teaching is a very important component of preoperative care, it is not considered essential baseline data.
   (Page 809)

5. **CORRECT ANSWER IS 4**
   The nurse's responsibility for teaching includes the type of equipment the patient may require postoperatively. The other explanations are provided by the physician with reinforcement by the nurse.
   (Page 810)

6. **CORRECT ANSWER IS 2**
   The scrub starts at the incision site and moves toward the periphery.
   (Page 816)

7. **CORRECT ANSWER IS 1**
   Previous surgeries do not necessarily place the patient at risk. The surgical history relevant to complications would be important to review to determine the risk state.
   (Page 817)

8. CORRECT ANSWER IS 4
Some facilities may include this information; however, the other three factors are necessary as major safety factors for the perioperative period.
(Page 819)

9. CORRECT ANSWER IS 4
The surgeon's signature is not required on the consent form. His name appears on the form, but he does not usually sign it.
(Page 818)

10. CORRECT ANSWER IS 3
The patient's history should not be repeated in the preoperative care charting. It is found in the admission data section of the chart.
(Page 820)

11. CORRECT ANSWER IS 3
Food and fluids are withheld until bowel sounds are present. This prevents abdominal distention, vomiting, and perhaps paralytic ileus.
(Page 825)

12. CORRECT ANSWER IS 3
The temperature usually reaches 102°F within the first 48 hours postoperatively.
(Page 826)

Chapter Twenty-Nine
Patient Education and Discharge Planning

QUESTIONS

1. Many patients experience resistance to change in the learning process. An important barrier that may be causing this resistance is

   1. Fear of change.
   2. Poor concentration.
   3. Age.
   4. Sex.

2. Which of the following is considered a risk factor requiring discharge planning?

   1. Middle-age group.
   2. Occupation.
   3. A chronic or terminal illness.
   4. Stable living arrangement.

3. The primary purpose of patient education is to

   1. Collect patient data.
   2. Determine readiness to learn.
   3. Assess degree of compliance.
   4. Increase patient's knowledge that will affect health status.

4. Patient teaching includes, in order, collecting patient data, determining readiness to learn, identifying patient learning needs, and _____.

   1. Evaluating results
   2. Determining appropriate teaching strategy
   3. Charting progress
   4. Assessing teaching situation

5. An important component of a discharge plan is

   1. Discharge charting.
   2. Information.
   3. Goal achievement.
   4. Short- and long-term goals.

6. Included as part of your responsibility in preparing your patient for discharge is to

   1. Obtain the medications the patient will take home.
   2. Evaluate the degree to which the patient education plan was implemented.
   3. Discuss with the family the pros and cons of discharge.
   4. Ask the patient if he is ready for discharge.

ANSWERS

1. CORRECT ANSWER IS 1
   Perceived threat or fear of change is a major barrier to change and may interrupt the teaching process.
   (Page 836)

2. CORRECT ANSWER IS 3
   A person with a chronic or terminal illness will be in a high-risk group that requires discharge planning. Other factors are elderly age, financial insecurity, inappropriate living arrangement, and so on.
   (Page 838)

3. **CORRECT ANSWER IS 4**
Purposes include increasing knowledge, increasing self-esteem, improving patient's ability to make decisions, and facilitating behavioral changes.
(Page 839)

4. **CORRECT ANSWER IS 2**
After the initial three steps, it is time to determine teaching strategy before evaluating results and charting progress.
(Page 841)

5. **CORRECT ANSWER IS 4**
The most specific answer is goals, both short- and long-term. Goal achievement is on the discharge summary.
(Page 845)

6. **CORRECT ANSWER IS 2**
It is part of your responsibility to evaluate the effectiveness of the patient education plan and reinforce those aspects that were incomplete or at least refer them to the home agency. The other answers are not your responsibility.
(Page 845)

Chapter Thirty
Crisis and the Dying Patient

QUESTIONS

1. A crisis can occur as a result of several factors including the visit of a loved one.
   1. True.
   2. False.

2. Crisis occurs as a result of an inability to cope with a situation, even though feelings of loss of control do not occur.
   1. True.
   2. False.

3. The third stage in the grief process as described by George Engle is
   1. Awareness.
   2. Idealization.
   3. Restitution.
   4. Resolution.

4. A patient with the diagnosis of cancer of the liver says, "Oh, there's nothing really wrong with me. I've just been working hard." This reaction, according to Elisabeth Kübler-Ross, is called
   1. Defense mechanism.
   2. Denial.
   3. Rationalization.
   4. Anxiety.

5. Elizabeth Kübler-Ross defines anger as the _____ phase of the grieving process
   1. First
   2. Second
   3. Third
   4. Fourth

6. Assisting a patient to handle a crisis situation involves setting firm limits and keeping the interaction goal-oriented.
   1. True.
   2. False.

7. "Marjorie, let's talk about how you are feeling now." This focus intervention by a crisis therapist is an example of
   1. Goal-oriented therapy.
   2. Insight therapy.
   3. Reality-oriented therapy.
   4. Focus therapy.

8. When a patient is in the denial phase of the grief process, diverting the conversation from happier times assists the patient to move into the anger stage.
   1. True.
   2. False.

9. To provide comfort and assistance to the dying patient, the nurse should always stay with him, even if he seems to withdraw and his actions indicate he wants to be alone.
   1. True.
   2. False.

10. Providing postmortem care includes all of the following actions EXCEPT
    1. Raising the head slightly.
    2. Placing dentures in the mouth.
    3. Cleansing the body.
    4. Removing all tubes and drains.

ANSWERS

1. CORRECT ANSWER IS 1
This is one factor causing a crisis situation. Others include marriage, unemployment, and loss of a loved one.
(Page 851)

2. CORRECT ANSWER IS 2
Crisis occurs as a result of loss of control and an inability to cope.
(Page 851)

3. CORRECT ANSWER IS 3
This is the ritual stage when initiation of the recovery process takes place.
(Page 852)

4. CORRECT ANSWER IS 2
The patient is experiencing denial—a temporary defense used as a buffer until the patient is able to face the implications of the diagnosis.
(Page 842)

5. CORRECT ANSWER IS 2
Anger follows denial in the grief process. In this stage a person is angry at having to give up life.
(Page 852)

6. CORRECT ANSWER IS 1
This action will keep the patient focused on the situation and active in problem-solving.
(Page 854)

7. CORRECT ANSWER IS 3
This statement is an example of "here and now" or reality-oriented therapy, a primary focus of crisis intervention.
(Page 854)

8. CORRECT ANSWER IS 2
It is essential to allow the patient to express himself by discussing happier times in order to progress to the other phases of the grief process.
(Page 857)

9. CORRECT ANSWER IS 2
The most appropriate assistance for a dying patient is to identify cues that indicate he wants privacy and to be alone.
(Page 860)

10. CORRECT ANSWER IS 4
Many facilities request that tubes and drains remain in the patient, especially if an autopsy is to be completed.
(Page 861)

Chapter Thirty-One
Advanced Skills in Nursing Practice

QUESTIONS

1. When performing defibrillation, the pads are usually placed
   1. Below the left clavicle at the midclavicular line and the 5th intercostal space, midclavicular line.
   2. Left anterior axillary line, 2nd intercostal space and the sternal border, right 2nd intercostal space.
   3. Right clavicle at sternoclavicular joint and left of cardiac apex, anterior axillary line.
   4. Right sternal border, 5th intercostal space and left of cardiac apex, anterior axillary line.

2. The machine is set to deliver 50 to 100 watt seconds for cardioversion.
   1. True.
   2. False.

3. When an external pacemaker is functioning correctly, all of the following actions will occur EXCEPT
   1. Artifact will be present either before the QRS complex or preceding the P wave.
   2. Pace/sense needle is constant and in the middle of the dial.
   3. MA output dial is set above 0.1 milliamperes.
   4. Rate/RPM will be set according to physician's orders.

4. After removing an arterial line, you need to apply pressure to the arterial site for at least 10 minutes.
   1. True.
   2. False.

5. When balancing the transducer, what reading will indicate it is balanced to atmospheric pressure?
   1. 0.
   2. 50.
   3. 100.
   4. 300.

6. The transducer is positioned at the level of the right ventricle to ensure an accurate reading.
   1. True.
   2. False.

7. The pressure alarm is activated on the ventilator. What is the most appropriate initial nursing action?
   1. Check for obstructions in tubing.
   2. Discontinue ventilator and hand ventilate.
   3. Check for disconnected tubing.
   4. Deflate and reinflate the airway cuff.

8. If a tension pneumothorax occurs, you should be prepared to immediately
   1. Assist the physician with chest tube insertion.
   2. Assist physician or perform chest decompression with a large-bore needle.
   3. Discontinue the ventilator and extubate the patient.
   4. Draw ABGs.

9. When taking a patient off ventilator therapy, you expect a slight increase in blood pressure and pulse.
   1. True.
   2. False.

ANSWERS

1. CORRECT ANSWER IS 3
This placement is used to provide a countershock which depolarizes all the cells simultaneously.
(Page 870)

2. CORRECT ANSWER IS 2
The machine delivers 25 to 50 watt seconds for cardioversion.
(Page 871)

3. CORRECT ANSWER IS 2
The pace/sense needle deflects to the right when the pacemaker is functioning accurately.
(Page 880)

4. CORRECT ANSWER IS 2
Pressure must be applied for 5 minutes.
(Page 890)

5. CORRECT ANSWER IS 1
Balancing the transducer ensures a more accurate reading.
(Page 899)

6. CORRECT ANSWER IS 2
The right atrium is the level at which the transducer is positioned.
(Page 899)

7. CORRECT ANSWER IS 1
When tubing is obstructed, pressure increases in the system triggering the sensitive alarm.
(Page 907)

8. CORRECT ANSWER IS 2
This must be done immediately to preserve function of the remaining lung.
(Page 908)

9. CORRECT ANSWER IS 1
You would expect a change in vital signs as the patient is weaned. Anxiety may also increase during this period.
(Page 910)

Chapter Thirty-Two
Home Care

QUESTIONS

1. A smooth transition from hospital to home depends on
   1. Discharge from the hospital when the patient is independent.
   2. Adequate physician instructions to the family.
   3. Appropriate discharge plan.
   4. Complete patient teaching while in hospital.

2. Health care documents for patients being cared for by a Home Health facility include admission sheet, progress sheet, and Patient Care Plan.
   1. True.
   2. False.

3. The nurse must visit at the same time as the home health aide to observe care and discuss the plan of care at least every 14 days.
   1. True.
   2. False.

4. To receive home care coverage from Medicare, the patient must be homebound. This means the patient's condition severely restricts leaving the home.
   1. True.
   2. False.

5. Nondisposable equipment can be sterilized by boiling the equipment in
   1. Prepared normal saline solution.
   2. A pan with 1/4" tap water.
   3. Water for 20 minutes.
   4. Jar containing tap water.

6. When teaching a home care patient, you should emphasize the signs that indicate pacemaker malfunction. These include
   1. Increased urine output.
   2. Regular, slow pulse.
   3. Weakness, fatigue.
   4. Disorientation.

ANSWERS

1. CORRECT ANSWER IS 3
   A discharge plan provides information on nursing procedures, medications, and equipment needed for care. This ensures that care is provided similarly in both settings.
   (Page 918)

2. CORRECT ANSWER IS 1
   These three documents include all of the relevant information (such as vital signs, discharge plan, and so on).
   (Page 920)

3. CORRECT ANSWER IS 2
   The nurse must visit the patient with the aide every 28 days.
   (Page 920)

4. CORRECT ANSWER IS 1
   This definition implies that it will be very difficult for the patient to leave home; for example, the patient requires assistance of another person or special transportation.
   (Page 921)

5. CORRECT ANSWER IS 3
Less time may not be sufficient for sterilization.
(Page 929)

6. CORRECT ANSWER IS 3
These symptoms indicate hypoxia to tissues.
(Page 950)

Section II Study Exercises

Chapter One
Professional Nursing

QUESTIONS

1. Define what is meant by the terms accountable and responsible when referring to the professional role of the nurse.

2. Define the following terms.

   A. Negligence

   B. Malpractice

   C. Liability

3. Discuss the concept of Universal Precautions.

4. List five precautions to prevent transmission of HIV.

   A.

   B.

   C.

   D.

   E.

ANSWERS

1. Review content on page 2: Professional Role.

2. Review content on page 6: The Elements of Liability.

3. Review content on page 13: Application of Universal Precautions.

4. Review content on page 14: Precautions to Prevent Transmission of HIV.

Chapter Two
Nursing Process

QUESTIONS

1. Define the PES framework for Nursing Diagnosis.

P

E

S

2. List two nursing diagnoses under the following Patterns of Nursing Diagnosis approved by NANDA.

A. Exchanging

(1)

(2)

B. Relating

(1)

(2)

C. Moving

(1)

(2)

ANSWERS

1. Review content on page 26: A Framework for Nursing Diagnosis.

2. Review content on page 27.

Chapter Three
Patient Care Management

QUESTIONS

1. List four principles of delegation that promote safe, effective management of patient care.

   A.

   B.

   C.

   D.

2. List at least six activities you will include in a time management plan for delivering patient care.

   A.

   B.

   C.

   D.

   E.

   F.

3. Describe at least four categories of data included on a Clinical Prep sheet.

   A.

   B.

   C.

   D.

4. Prepare a Patient Care Plan using the format on page 31 (Figure 3–2). Develop one nursing diagnosis, no more than two expected outcomes, and three or four nursing interventions. Use a nursing diagnosis from *Pattern 1: Exchanging*.

   Patient scenario for the care plan:

   James Brown, a 68-year-old retired coal miner, has been diagnosed with chronic obstructive pulmonary disease. He is admitted to the medical nursing unit with right lower lobe pneumonia.

ANSWERS

1. Review content on pages 37–38: General Principles of Delegation.

2. Review content on page 41: Time Management.

3. Review Prep Sheet on page 39.

4. Review content on pages 31–32: Care Plan.

    Nursing diagnosis should be one of the following:
    Impaired Gas Exchange
    Ineffective Airway Clearance
    Ineffective Breathing Pattern

    Expected Outcomes:
    Absence of adventitious breath sounds.
    Decrease in adventitious breath sounds.
    Respirations within normal range.
    Lungs clear to auscultation.

    Interventions: See page 32, Figure 3–4.

Chapter Four
Documentation

QUESTIONS

1. List five rules for charting narrative notes in source-oriented narrative charting.

   A.

   B.

   C.

   D.

   E.

2. Define what is meant by a "problem" in problem-oriented medical records.

3. Define the following.

   A. ad lib

   B. b.i.d.

   C. hemi

   D. lb.

   E. n.p.o.

   F. p.c.

   G. q.h.

   H. s

ANSWERS

1. Review content on pages 51–53: Source-Oriented Narrative Charting.

2. Review content on page 55: Problem-Oriented Medical Records.

3. Review content on pages 68–69: Word Roots, Prefixes, and Suffixes.

Chapter Five
Communication and Relationship Skills

QUESTIONS

1. List and define three therapeutic communication techniques.

A.

B.

C.

2. List the phases in a nurse–patient relationship.

A.

B.

C.

ANSWERS

1. Review content on pages 73–75: Therapeutic Communication Techniques.

2. Review content on page 77: Phases in Nurse–Patient Relationship Therapy.

Chapter Six
Safe Patient Environment

QUESTIONS

1. List one nursing diagnosis with related factors/risk factors.

   A. Nursing Diagnosis:

   B. Related or risk factors:

2. Discuss one potential problem related to skin care and give two possible solutions.

   A. Potential problem:

   B. Possible solutions:
   (1)

   (2)

ANSWERS

1. Review content on page 98: Nursing Diagnoses.

2. Review content on page 106.

Chapter Seven
Bathing and Bedmaking

QUESTIONS

1. List three principles of medical asepsis.

    A.

    B.

    C.

2. Discuss two nursing actions necessary to prevent skin breakdown.

    A.

    B.

ANSWERS

1. Review content on page 122: Medical Asepsis.

2. Review content on page 132: Preventing Skin Breakdown.

Chapter Eight
Personal Hygiene

QUESTIONS

1. Define the following terms.

　A. Canthus

　B. Excoriation

　C. Nasolacrimal

　D. Pediculosis

　E. Thrush

2. Describe how you would drape a female patient before providing perineal care.

3. List at least four assessment parameters for oral hygiene.

　A.

　B.

　C.

　D.

4. Describe at least four common foot problems.

　A.

　B.

　C.

　D.

5. State three nursing diagnoses that are appropriate to include in a patient care plan for hygienic care interventions.

　A.

　B.

　C.

ANSWERS

1. Review definitions on pages 166–167.
2. Review content on page 159.
3. Review page 146: Assessment Data Base for Oral Hygiene.
4. Review content on page 145: Foot Care.
5. Review content on pages 145–146: Nursing Diagnosis.

Chapter Nine
Vital Signs

QUESTIONS

1. Explain how the following factors affect blood pressure.

   A. Cardiac output

   B. Peripheral vascular resistance

   C. Blood viscosity

   D. Chemoreceptors

2. Define the following phases of Korotkoff Sounds.

   A. Phase I

   B. Phase III

   C. Phase V

3. List four possible sites for determining pulse rate.

   A.

   B.

   C.

   D.

4. Describe the difference between Cheyne-Stokes and Kussmaul's respirations.

ANSWERS

1. Review content on page 175: Blood Pressure.

2. Review content on page 176: Korotkoff Sounds.

3. Review content from pages 183–186; see illustration on page 184.

4. Review content on page 200: Respiratory Terminology and note illustration on page 190.

Chapter Ten
Body Mechanics and Positioning

QUESTIONS

1. List four guidelines that are important for implementation of body mechanics.

    A.

    B.

    C.

    D.

2. Fill in the steps of using Basic Principles to move an object by pushing and pulling to expend minimal energy.

    A. Stand close to the object.

    B. _____

    C. Tense muscles and prepare for movement.

    D. _____

    E. Push away from you by leaning toward object using body weight to add force.

ANSWERS

1. Review content on page 203: Body Mechanics.

2. Review content on page 205: Using Basic Principles.

Chapter Eleven
Exercise and Ambulation

QUESTIONS

1. Define the following terms.

   A. Antagonist muscles

   B. Synergistic muscles

   C. Synarthrotic joints

   D. Diarthrotic joints

2. Write three nursing diagnoses that would be appropriate to use for a patient needing assistance with exercise and ambulation.

   A.

   B.

   C.

3. Describe how you would teach quadricep-setting and gluteal-setting exercises to a patient.

4. Briefly describe how to accurately measure a patient for crutches.

5. Describe two actions you would use if a patient complains of numbness and tingling in fingers when crutch walking.

   A.

   B.

6. After instructing a patient on crutch walking, you would chart the following information:

ANSWERS

1. Review the content on pages 223–224: Muscle Function.

2. Review content on page 226: Nursing Diagnosis.

3. Review content on page 237: Teaching Muscle-Strengthening Exercises.

4. Review content on pages 237–238: Measuring Patient for Crutches.

5. Review content on page 241: Clinical Problem Solving.

6. Review content on page 241: Charting for Crutch Walking.

Chapter Twelve
Admission and Discharge

QUESTIONS

1. Discuss the rationale for informing patients of the *Patient's Bill of Rights*.

2. List two factors related to the nursing diagnosis of *Grieving, Anticipatory*.

   A.

   B.

3. Discuss two suggested solutions for correcting the problem of a patient's weight varying excessively from one day to the next.

   A.

   B.

ANSWERS

1. Refer to content on page 245: Admission to the Nursing Unit.

2. Review content on page 247: Nursing Diagnosis.

3. Review content on page 254: Clinical Problem Solving.

Chapter Thirteen
Basic Physical Assessment

QUESTIONS

1. List the primary equipment you will have available to complete a physical assessment on a patient.

   A.

   B.

   C.

   D.

   E.

2. Discuss four elements of a health history.

   A.

   B.

   C.

   D.

3. Describe the difference between decorticate and decerebrate posturing and suggest a possible lesion site for each one.

4. Fill in the following blanks for pupil assessment.

	Normal	Abnormal
Size of pupils	Diameter 1.5–6 mm	_____
		_____
Shape of pupils	Round and midposition	_____
		_____
Equality of pupils	_____	Unequal—sign that parasympathetic and sympathetic nervous systems are not synchronized.
Light reflex	Pupil constricts	_____

5. Complete the following sentences

   A. Discontinuous sounds: Rales are due to _____

   B. Continuous sounds: Rhonchi are produced by _____

   C. Wheezes are produced by _____

121

6. Differentiate between assessing S_1 heart sounds and S_2 heart sounds.

7. When assessing urine output, the normal findings are

   A. Output

   B. Color

   C. Odor

   D. Specific gravity

   E. pH range

8. List two questions that will help you assess the patient's mental status in terms of thought process and perception.

   A.

   B.

ANSWERS

1. Refer to content on page 262: Types of Equipment.

2. Refer to content on page 263: Health History.

3. Review content on pages 263–264: Level of Consciousness.

4. Review content on pages 264–265: Pupil Assessment.

5. Review content on page 279: Lung Sounds.

6. Review content on page 280: Heart Assessment.

7. Review content on page 284: Urinary Tract Assessment.

8. Review content on page 287: Thought Processes and Perception.

Chapter Fourteen
Infection Control and AIDS Care

QUESTIONS

1. Describe the three ways in which the body resists infection.

   A.

   B.

   C.

2. State the three requirements for double-bagging isolation items.

   A.

   B.

   C.

3. Discuss precautions for disposing of the following.

   A. Secretions

   B. Excretions

   C. Blood

4. You are drawing blood from an HIV positive patient when you accidentally get blood in your eye and on your arms. Your immediate nursing interventions include

123

ANSWERS

1. Review content on page 292: Barriers to Infection.

2. Review content on page 307: Three Requirements for Double-Bagging.

3. Review content on page 308: Clinical Alert for Disposal Precautions.

4. Review content on page 314: Clinical Problem Solving.

Chapter Fifteen
Medication Administration

QUESTIONS

1. Fill in the missing steps of drug metabolism.

   A. Absorption

   B. _____

   C. Biotransformation

   D. _____

2. Safety procedures are important when administering drugs. List the "Five Rights" or safety rules of medication administration.

   A.

   B.

   C.

   D.

   E.

3. The physician's order is to give 750 mg of Penicillin. Dose on hand is capsules—250 mg. You will give _____ capsules.

4. List two suggestions that will help children accept their medications more readily.

   A.

   B.

5. Describe the missing steps of combining medications in one syringe with two vials.

   A. Prepare both vials by _____ tops.

   B. Inject air from syringe into _____ vial.

   C. Inject air from syringe into _____ vial.

   D. Invert vial and withdraw ordered amount of medication from _____ vial.

   E. Insert needle, invert and withdraw ordered amount of medication from _____ vial.

6. List the steps of TBC testing.

   A.

   B.

   C.

7. Discuss the nursing action indicated if you are assigned to administer a heparin injection and the partial thromboplastin (PTT) is double the control time.

125

8. List two rationales for *not* massaging the area following a heparin injection.

   A.

   B.

9. The peak action time of regular insulin is _____, while the peak action time of NPH is _____. Long-acting insulin (protamine zinc and ultralente) have an onset time of _____ and duration time of _____.

10. List three techniques for minimizing pain during injections.

    A.

    B.

    C.

ANSWERS

1. Review content on pages 318–319: Drug Metabolism.

2. Review content on page 320: Safety Procedures.

3. Refer to the formula on page 324: Converting Medications.

4. Review procedure on page 330: Administering Oral Medications to Children.

5. Review procedure on page 336: Combining Medications in One Syringe Using Two Vials.

6. Review content on page 338: TBC Testing.

7. Review content on page 339: Clinical Alert for Heparin Injection.

8. Review content on page 340: Administering SubQ Heparin.

9. Review Insulin Chart on page 340: Insulin Types and Action.

10. Review box on page 346: Techniques for Minimizing Pain During Injections.

Chapter Sixteen
Pain Management

QUESTIONS

1. Briefly describe the Gate Control Theory.

2. When considering how pain manifests in the body, fill in the blank lines with a description of the characteristics of pain.

   A. Location

      1. _____

      2. _____

   B. Quality of pain

      1. _____

      2. _____

   C. Intensity

      1. _____

   D. Physiological factors associated with pain

      1. _____

      2. _____

      3. _____

   E. Precipitating factors

      1. _____

      2. _____

   F. Aggravating factors

      1. _____

      2. _____

   G. Alleviating factors

      1. _____

      2. _____

3. The rationale for requiring special certification for administering narcotics via an indwelling epidural catheter is

4. List three criteria for patient selection for Patient Controlled Analgesia (PCA).

   A.

   B.

   C.

ANSWERS

1. Review content on page 368: Gate Control Theory.

2. Refer to content on page 371: Characteristics of Pain.

3. Review content on page 377: see box for Administering Epidural Narcotic Analgesia.

4. Refer to page 380: Criteria for Patient Selection PCA.

Chapter Seventeen
Nutritional Management

QUESTIONS

1. List the six essential nutrients necessary for sustaining life.

    A.

    B.

    C.

    D.

    E.

    F.

2. List three foods that are restricted on a low-calcium diet.

    A.

    B.

    C.

3. A low-purine diet is suggested for a patient with the diagnosis of _____ _____.

4. You are assigned to administer an intermittent nasogastric feeding. You aspirate stomach contents and it is 100 mL. The appropriate nursing intervention is to

ANSWERS

1. Review content on page 392: Essential Nutrients.

2. Refer to information on page 404: Low-calcium Diet.

3. Review content on page 404: Low-purine Diet.

4. Refer to the skill on page 410: Giving an Intermittent Nasogastric Feeding.

Chapter Eighteen
Specimen Collection

QUESTIONS

1. Write two nursing diagnoses that can be used for patients requiring specimen collection.

A.

B.

2. Define the following terms.

A. Aerobe

B. Anaerobe

C. Autolet

D. Culture

ANSWERS

1. Review content on page 430: Nursing Diagnosis.

2. Review content on page 448: Terminology.

Chapter Nineteen
Diagnostic Tests

QUESTIONS

1. List four symptoms associated with reactions to contrast media.

   A.

   B.

   C.

   D.

2. Describe at least five factors that are charted for patients undergoing diagnostic procedures.

   A.

   B.

   C.

   D.

   E.

3. If a patient complains of dyspnea following a thoracentesis, your priority interventions include

   A.

   B.

   C.

ANSWERS

1. Review content on page 456: Clinical Alert.

2. Review content on page 472: Charting for Diagnostic Procedures.

3. Review content on page 473: Clinical Problem Solving.

Chapter Twenty
Urine Elimination

QUESTIONS

1. Explain the process of micturition.

2. There are several alterations that occur in urinary elimination. Give one example for each alteration. *Example:* Alteration Related to Fluids–Decrease in fluid intake.

    A. Alteration Related to Secretion of the Antidiuretic Hormone–

    B. Alterations Related to Changes in Blood Volume–

3. Discuss the difference between the 5-drop and 2-drop method for the Clinitest.

4. You are monitoring your patient's status during the cycle of peritoneal dialysis. List four important parameters to assess for during the cycle.

    A.

    B.

    C.

    D.

ANSWERS

1. Review content on page 478: Micturition.

2. Refer to content on page 479: Alterations in Urinary Elimination.

3. Refer to the skill on pages 484–485: Measuring Urine Glucose.

4. Review content on page 512: Maintaining Peritoneal Dialysis.

Chapter Twenty-One
Bowel Elimination

QUESTIONS

1. Compare a colostomy and ileostomy for the following factors.

	Colostomy	Ileostomy
A. Surgical Procedure	_____	_____
B. Bowel Control	_____	_____
C. Stool Consistency	_____	_____
D. Diet Control	_____	_____

2. List one type of enema for each category.

Category	Type
A. Cleansing	_____
B. Retention	_____
C. Distention Reduction	_____
D. Medicated	_____

ANSWERS

1. Review Table 21–1 on page 531: Comparison Chart for Ostomies.

2. Review content on page 539.

Chapter Twenty-Two
Heat and Cold Therapy

QUESTIONS

1. State the assessment data necessary when moist heat is applied to a patient.

   A.

   B.

   C.

   D.

2. Complete the following chart.

Application	Use	Precautions
Heat Lamp		
Aquathermic Pad		
Heat Cradle		

3. If a patient's skin becomes macerated while using the cooling blanket, you should perform the following nursing interventions.

   A.

   B.

4. An appropriate Nursing Diagnosis for a patient requiring hot or cold treatment is

ANSWERS

1. Review content on page 562: Assessment Data Base.

2. Review content on page 568: Table 22–1, Dry Heat Application.

3. Review content on page 574: Clinical Problem Solving.

4. Review content on page 561: Pain or Skin Integrity, Impaired.

Chapter Twenty-Three
Wound Care

QUESTIONS

1. Define the following terms.

    A. Primary healing

    B. Second intention

2. List three preventive steps for avoiding pressure ulcers in high-risk patients.

    A.

    B.

    C.

3. List the related factors or risk factors for the nursing diagnosis of Skin Integrity, Impaired.

    A.

    B.

    C.

4. Compare and contrast the procedure for cleaning a clean wound and a dirty wound.

	Clean Wound	Dirty Wound
A. Size pad		
B. Cleansing procedure		
C. Discard procedure		

5. Discuss the rationale for using different wet dressings.

Type of Dressing	Purpose
Wet-to-damp	
Wet-to-dry	
Wet-to-wet	

6. Describe the staging of pressure ulcers.

   A. Stage 1

   B. Stage 2

   C. Stage 3

   D. Stage 4

ANSWERS

1. Refer to content on page 582: Wound Healing.

2. Review content on page 584: Pressure Ulcers.

3. Refer to the Nursing Diagnosis section, page 585: Skin Integrity, Impaired.

4. Review content on page 593: Clinical Alert for Clean and Dirty Wounds.

5. Refer to the chart on page 603: Wet Dressings.

6. Review content on page 605: Pressure Ulcer Staging.

Chapter Twenty-Four
Respiratory Care

QUESTIONS

1. State three Nursing Diagnoses and their associated related factors for patients who require respiratory assistance.

    A.

    B.

    C.

2. Describe at least four clinical manifestations that must be assessed for patients requiring suctioning.

    A.

    B.

    C.

    D.

3. Four indications that a patient needs suctioning are

    A.

    B.

    C.

    D.

4. Complete the following chart by writing the size of suction catheter for

    A. Adults _____ French

    B. Children _____ French

    C. Infants _____ French

5. Early signs and symptoms of hypoxia include

    A.

    B.

    C.

    D.

6. List four advantages of pulse oximetry.

A.

B.

C.

D.

7. Compare and contrast the differences in nursing care for patient with a SCOOP 1 and SCOOP 2 catheter.

8. Describe the function of each bottle in the 3-bottle water seal system.

Function

Bottle #1

Bottle #2

Bottle #3

9. Describe the four principles of the water-seal system.

A.

B.

C.

D.

ANSWERS

1. Review content on page 614: Nursing Diagnosis.

2. Review content on page 623: Nursing Process Data.

3. Review content on page 624: Indications for Suctioning.

4. Answers: Adults 12–18; Children 8–10; Infants 5–8 (Page 626).

5. Review content on page 629: Symptoms of Hypoxia.

6. Review content on page 631: Why Pulse Oximetry?

7. Review content on page 639: Providing Catheter Care.

8. Review content on page 659: Bottle Systems.

9. Review content on page 660: Principles of the Water-Seal System.

Chapter Twenty-Five
Circulatory Maintenance

QUESTIONS

1. List at least six generalized signs and symptoms for hemorrhaging.

   A.

   B.

   C.

   D.

   E.

   F.

2. State two nursing diagnoses with related factors that can be incorporated in a patient care plan for a patient with circulatory impairment.

   Nursing Diagnoses **Related Factors**
   A.   A.

   B.   B.

3. Describe charting parameters for patients requiring Sequential Compression Devices.

   A.

   B.

   C.

   D.

4. An appropriate nursing intervention when ECG electrodes do not adhere to the skin is to

ANSWERS

1. Review content on page 678: Table 25–1, Assessment Guide for Hemorrhaging.

2. Review content on page 679: Nursing Diagnosis.

3. Review charting on page 686: For Compression Devices.

4. One of the following interventions can be used to adhere ECG electrodes to the skin (Page 691):
   1. Change placement of electrodes.
   2. Use Tincture of Benzoin on skin.
   3. Cleanse skin with alcohol swab.

Chapter Twenty-Six
Intravenous Therapy

QUESTIONS

1. List the major electrolytes and their symbols.

Cations	Symbol
A.	
B.	
C.	
D.	

Anions	Symbol
E.	
F.	
G.	

2. Discuss two reasons for the current practice of using IV filters for IV administration.

   A.

   B.

3. List three criteria for selecting a vein in preparation for IV administration.

   A.

   B.

   C.

4. Discuss the primary advantage of using a through-the-needle catheter rather than an over-the-needle catheter.

5. IV calorie calculation. Fill in the blanks.

   A. 2000 mL D_5W provides _____ g of dextrose.

   B. 100 g of dextrose provides _____ calories.

   C. 2000 mL provides _____ calories.

   D. Usual IV total/day is _____ mL, which will provide _____ calories.

6. When establishing IV administration, would you choose to use a controller or pump? Give the rationale for your choice.

7. For each complication of IV therapy listed below, suggest two nursing interventions.

   A. Phlebitis
   1.

   2.

   B. Infiltration
   1.

   2.

   C. Air embolism
   1.

   2.

   D. Infection at site
   1.

   2.

   E. Allergic reaction
   1.

   2.

8. List four signs of dehydration that you would assess for when you are completing a physical assessment on a patient who has been lost in the wilderness for 4 days.

   A.

   B.

   C.

   D.

9. Fill in the change that occurs in vital signs when a person is excessively hydrated or dehydrated.

	Excess Hydration	Dehydration
A. Blood Pressure		
B. Pulse		
C. Temperature		
D. Respirations		

10. Discuss the primary difference between the Hickman or Broviac CV catheter and the Groshong CV catheter.

ANSWERS

1. Review content on page 704: Table 26–2, Major Electrolytes.

2. Refer to "boxed" content on page 706: IV Filters.

3. Review content on page 711: Preparing IV Site–Procedure.

4. Review content on page 716: Inserting a Through-the-Needle Catheter.

5. Refer to "boxed" content on page 718: IV Calorie Calculation.

6. Review content on page 719: Choice: Controller or Pump.

7. Refer to content on page 724: Clinical Alert–Complications of IV Therapy.

8. Review content on Dehydration, page 729: Table 26–3, Body Sites for Assessment of Hydration.

9. Refer to chart on page 729: Table 26–4, Objective Data Indicative of the State of Hydration.

10. Review content on pages 752–755: note the Clinical Alert on page 755.

Chapter Twenty-Seven
Orthopedic Measures

QUESTIONS

1. Briefly define the different types of fractures listed below.

   A. Greenstick

   B. Comminuted

   C. Open or compound

   D. Closed or simple

   E. Compression

2. Match the type of traction in Column A with the definition in Column B.

Column A	Column B
____ 1. Bryant's traction	A. Applied for short periods of time; commonly used for knee injuries.
____ 2. Buck's traction	B. Russell's and Thomas splint with Pearson attachment.
____ 3. Skeletal traction	C. Used primarily for children.
____ 4. Types of skeletal traction	D. Maintains reduction of the fractured limb.

3. Visualize applying a figure-eight bandage on a friend's sprained ankle and write the procedure step-by-step.

   A. Anchor bandage around distal end of foot.

   B.

   C.

   D.

   E. Complete wrapping by covering area above and below ankle.

4. List two advantages of the plaster cast over the synthetic cast.

   A.

   B.

5. List three interventions that will assist in preventing pin site infection for the Halo traction.

   A.

   B.

   C.

149

ANSWERS

1. Review content on pages 767–768: Types of Fractures.

2. Review content on page 768: Traction. Correct answers: 1=B, 2=D, 3=A, 4=C.

3. Review procedure on page 772: Applying a Figure-Eight Bandage.

4. Review content on page 776: Table 27–1, Comparison of Casts.

5. Refer to the procedure on page 783: Monitoring Halo Traction, #6.

Chapter Twenty-Eight
Operative Care

QUESTIONS

1. Many patients experience anxiety and stress when they anticipate surgery. List three factors that influence the degree of anxiety or stress that may be experienced.

   A.

   B.

   C.

2. Your assignment is to complete a Preoperative Stress Assessment. In each category below, list two possible responses indicating a high stress level.

   A. Physiological Responses
      1.

      2.

   B. Emotional Responses
      1.

      2.

   C. Anxiety Responses
      1.

      2.

3. List four types of patients at risk for postoperative infection.

   A.

   B.

   C.

   D.

4. If you are the nurse responsible for discharging a patient from the recovery room, which five criteria do you consider the most important?

   A.

   B.

   C.

   D.

   E.

5. List two preventative measures and two interventions for each of the postoperative complications listed below.

Potential Complication	Prevention Measure	Intervention
A. Atelectasis	1.	1.
	2.	2.
B. Pneumonia	1.	1.
	2.	2.
C. Thrombophlebitis	1.	1.
	2.	2.
D. Wound infection	1.	1.
	2.	2.

ANSWERS

1. Refer to content on page 803: Preoperative Anxiety.

2. Review content on page 806: Table 28–3, Preoperative Stress Assessment.

3. Review content on page 817: Patients at Risk for Postoperative Infection.

4. Review material on page 823: Discharging Patient from Recovery Room.

5. Review content on pages 827–830: Table 28–4, Postoperative Complications.

Chapter Twenty-Nine
Patient Education and Discharge Planning

QUESTIONS

1. List two barriers to change that a nurse must confront during the patient education process. Suggest an approach to deal with the barriers.

        Barrier   Nursing Approach

A.

B.

2. Discuss the student nurse's role in patient education.

3. List three members of the health team that are important to provide a multidisciplinary approach for discharge planning.

A.

B.

C.

4. You are responsible for determining a teaching strategy for a patient newly diagnosed with diabetes who requires daily insulin injections.

Choose which type of teaching strategy will be most effective in this situation.

List three appropriate teaching adjuncts for this plan.

A.

B.

C.

5. Write examples of nursing actions or patient behavior for the components of a discharge summary listed below.

A. Document one example of psychosocial assessment.

B. Identify activity level of patient.

C. Describe use of a piece of equipment patient will require at home.

D. Describe two goals achieved in patient education.

E. Identify a referral agency.

F. Document two discharge instructions provided to family.

G. Describe method of discharge.

ANSWERS

1. Review content on page 836: Resistance to Change.

2. Refer to content on page 837: Student Nurse's Role in Patient Education.

3. Review content on page 838: Discharge Planning.

4. Review content on page 841: Determining Appropriate Teaching Strategy.

5. Review content on page 845: Completing a Discharge Summary.

Chapter Thirty
Crisis and the Dying Patient

QUESTIONS

1. Compare the *Stages of Grief* (George Engle) with the *Stages of Dying* (Elisabeth Kübler-Ross).

2. Discuss the purpose of a "Living Will."

3. If you are caring for a dying patient and find that you cannot cope with your own feelings about death, what is an appropriate resolution to this dilemma?

ANSWERS

1. Refer to content on pages 851–852: Stages of Grief, Stages of Dying.

2. Refer to content on page 859: Living Will.

3. Refer to content on page 860: Assisting the Dying Patient and Clinical Problem Solving.

Chapter Thirty-One
Advanced Skills in Nursing Practice

QUESTIONS

1. State a rationale for familiarizing all personnel with the emergency cart contents.

2. A defibrillator functions in a nonsynchronized mode, while cardioversion functions in a synchronized mode. Discuss this statement.

3. List three modes of temporary pacemaker therapy.
   A.
   B.
   C.

4. List three signs of pacemaker failure.
   A.
   B.
   C.

5. Complete the following sentences.
   A. The purpose of Allen's test is to
   B. This test is administered before beginning the procedure of

6. Discuss the difference between PEEP and CPAP as therapy.

ANSWERS

1. Review content on page 868: Using the Emergency Cart.

2. Refer to content on page 870: Performing Defibrillation.

3. Review content on pages 876–877: Pacemaker.

4. Refer to content on page 880: Clinical Alert.

5. Refer to content on page 885: Performing Allen's Test.

6. Refer to content on page 902: Airway Pressure Therapies.

Chapter Thirty-Two
Home Care

QUESTIONS

1. List four members of the Health Care Provider team with one major responsibility for each member.

          Team Member   **Responsibility**

A.

B.

C.

D.

2. Home care visits must be accurately documented for both _____ and _____ purposes.

3. List five major assessment areas that are necessary to determine safety in the home environment.

A.

B.

C.

D.

E.

4. If you are assigned to make a home visit, which guideline do you think is most important to follow for your home visit?

159

ANSWERS

1. Refer to content on page 917: Home Health Team.

2. Refer to content on page 919: Documentation.

3. Refer to content on pages 924–925: Assessing Home for Safe Environment.

4. Refer to content on page 924: Guidelines for Home Care.